Building
a Healthy
America

BUILDING A HEALTHY AMERICA

Conquering Disease and Disability

TERRY L. LIERMAN, Editor

Facts, Figures & Funding

Mary Ann Liebert, Inc. publishers

Copyright © 1987 by Capitol Associates Inc., 426 C Street, N.E., Washington, DC 20002

Published by Mary Ann Liebert, Inc., publishers, 1651 Third Avenue, New York, NY 10128

ISBN 0-913-113-12-3

Printed in the United States of America

To Mary Lasker,
a woman whose mind rebels
against needless suffering
and whose heart responds
to a worthy cause

Special thanks are extended
to the following organizations,
without whose support
this book would not have been possible:

The National Center for Health Education

The Commonwealth Fund

Merck Sharp & Dohme
Division of Merck & Co., Inc.

The Upjohn Company

The Commonwealth Fund

The Commonwealth Fund was established as a philanthropic foundation in 1918 by Anna M. Harkness. The name "Commonwealth" is derived from Mrs. Harkness' wish that the fund's resources be used to enhance the "common good." The fund provides grants to a variety of individuals and organizations to identify and help meet society's long-term health care needs.

This book was supported by a grant from The Commonwealth Fund. In all cases, the statements made and the views expressed are those of Terry L. Lierman and do not reflect those of The Commonwealth Fund.

The National Center for Health Education

The National Center for Health Education (NCHE) played a vital role in the creation of *Building a Healthy America,* serving as editorial advisor and financial coordinator.

NCHE is a private, not-for-profit center with the goal of strengthening education for health nationwide. It was created in 1975 at the recommendation of a Presidential committee.

NCHE acts as an advocate of education for health to save lives and lower medical costs. Such education draws on the skills of professional health educators, volunteers, and experts from a broad cross-section of other professions, such as medicine, business, and the news media.

Because those who conduct education for health work in many different roles and settings, NCHE seeks to foster communication among them, with the goal of promoting the establishment of new programs, improving educators' skills, and encouraging the spread of innovations.

For further information about the National Center for Health Education and its programs, call or write:

The National Center for Health Education
30 East 29th Street
New York, NY 10016
(212) 689-1886

Contents

Preface

When Americans are asked hypothetically if they could be granted just one wish, they invariably wish for "good health."

If health, then, is so important to us, why is it not this nation's #1 priority? Our current national health policy consists of simply paying bills, restricting services, and constricting payment to health professionals. In essence, we have no national health policy.

Every year Americans pay enormous bills for their health care. We are currently spending $440,000,000,000 on the delivery of health care services to take care of those who are not healthy. Yet we are spending only $8,000,000,000 to find the cures and treatments that would alleviate illness or, more importantly, keep people healthy.

Too much for needles—too little for microscopes.

If a healthy America is to become a priority, we must fight for it. We must insist on escalating our efforts in the war against disease and disability. Adequate funding is absolutely essential in this battle. Today, we are barely waging a skirmish.

Mary Lasker, the force behind this book, has been this country's leading proponent of the benefits of medical research. In previous publications (*Killers and Cripplers*, 1968-1976), she presented impressive statistics about the numbers of Americans afflicted by the major diseases and disabilities and the staggering costs both to the individual and to the country. This book continues that tradition.

Building a Healthy America goes even further. Armed with the statistics, we must now lobby Congress and our presidential candidates to guarantee that our health will not be jeopardized by the lack of funding for medical research. It is extraordinary to note that in 18 months the Defense Department spends more on research and development than has been spent in the entire 100-year history of the National Institutes of Health.

For every dollar spent on medical research, $13 is saved in lost wages, health care costs, and productivity. For example, over 50 percent of those in nursing homes have Alzheimer's disease—the costs and human suffering that could be avoided by the cure or prevention of this tragic disease are staggering. That would be real cost containment and not the shallow policy edicts of cutting back services and payments.

The decaying infrastructure of the research community must have growth. To accomplish this, a public agenda is needed for facilities and equipment renewal, training researchers, and supporting applied research to apply the results of a strong basic research program.

Rather than seizing the opportunity for progress, we as a nation are allowing it to slip away because of short-sighted public policy that is more concerned with short-term projects and cash than long-term value and real progress for all of us.

The result is the stagnation of one of the nation's and the world's most valuable resources—its medical research capability. "You can't develop a strong country if the people are sick," Mrs. Lasker says frequently, emphasizing that health must be a leading priority in this country.

This is a very exciting time in the history of medicine. The potential of medical research has never been brighter, in part from the advances in genetic engineering, the development of more refined and highly sensitive diagnostic techniques, and new therapeutics. This growing potential and the subsequent benefits must not be impeded by the lack of funding. To assure our health, our family's health, and our country's health, we all have to take up the cause.

This book includes vital information to make all of us effective advocates for health: how the federal government works for health, how to lobby for health, what is the status of various diseases, and where you can go to get more information and help. It also provides information on Congress and the Congressmen and Senators whose support we must secure in our endeavor to conquer disease and disability.

Issues assume importance, movements gain momentum, and bills become laws when backed either by a significant number of people or by a number of significant people. When such people identify a national problem and act to correct it, changes in public policy occur. When you put down this book, pick up your pen.

A clear and present need exists for all Americans to engage in a winnable war against disease and disability. It may not be a call to arms, but rather away from them, in terms of this nation's priorities. Now more than ever before, we must communicate our concerns and request our elected officials to take the initiative to build a healthy America.

A Note on Statistics

The statistics reported in this book were gathered from various agencies of the federal government, such as the National Institutes of Health and the Alcohol, Drug Abuse, and Mental Health Administration, and the National Center for Health Education and various voluntary organizations. All figures used herein are the latest for which authoritative data were available in mid 1987.

Amassing the statistics was a long, arduous, and often frustrating process. Information gathering is an expensive endeavor for health agencies, and as budgets tighten, the organizations often must choose between the collection of numbers and the sponsorship of research. But statistics are vital tools in setting priorities, measuring success in fighting disease, and describing the size of a problem that must be dealt with.

There is an urgent need for increased government funding for up-to-date and accurate statistics to aid in our effort to conquer disease and disability.

Terry L. Lierman
Editor

Acknowledgments

The successful completion of this book depended on the efforts of many people. Any success that this book achieves through the information that it provides or the inspiration that it instills can be attributed to the work of many researchers, writers, and editors. Some efforts have been acknowledged directly, some have not, yet all contributions have been vital. Any errors, omissions, or lack of inspiration are solely my responsibility.

When Mary Lasker asked that this book be done, it was a matter of how. It is a direct result of the following people.

The immediate encouragement of Margaret Mahoney and Cynthia Woodcock at The Commonwealth Fund, along with Clarence Pearson, Stephanie Lederman, Bill Gross, and David Van Fossen at the National Center for Health Education really got this book on track. This was followed by generous support from Dr. Ted Cooper of The Upjohn Company and Tony Fiskett at Merck Sharp & Dohme, people I am lucky to call friends.

A more enthusiastic and helpful publisher an editor never had. Mary Ann Liebert and her staff, especially Vicki Cohn and Audrey Shepard, brought this book to fruition.

Any book on medical research could not be compiled without help from those who work with the programs at the National Institutes of Health and the Alcohol, Drug Abuse, and Mental Health Administration. People too numerous to mention get kudos, but Dr. Jay Moskowitz was particularly helpful, as were Dr. Bill Rhode, Ron Winterrowd, Joan Baily, Ed McManus, Dr. Murray Goldstein, Dr. Claude Lenfant, Diane Shartsis Wax, Dr. James Hill, Dr. Peter Frommer, and Dr. Ian MacDonald.

My colleagues at Capitol Associates, Inc., put more than their fair share of the work into this as well — Debra Hardy, a true partner, Linda Baumes, Weston Frank, Pamela Jackson, Marianne Lile, Gordon MacDougall, Wendy Noerr, Julie Rhea, and Frankie Trull.

The following organizations provided information for the compilation of statistics for this project: Alcohol, Drug Abuse, and Mental Health Administration (ADAMHA), Alzheimer's Disease and Related Disorders Association, American Academy of Otolaryngology—Head and Neck Surgery, American Cancer Society, American Diabetes Association, American Foundation for the Blind, American Heart Association, American Hospital Association, American Lung Association, American Optometric Association, American Psychiatric Association, American Psychological Association, American Speech-Language-Hearing Association, American Trauma Society, Arthritis Foundation, Center for Sickle Cell Disease, Howard University, Citizens for the Treatment of High Blood Pressure, Inc., Cystic Fibrosis Foundation, Food and Drug Administration, Foundation for Biomedical Research, High Blood Pressure Education Program—National Institutes of Health, Lupus Foundation of America, National Association of Rehabilitation Facilities, National Cancer Institute, National Council on Alcoholism, Inc., National Eye Institute, National Health Council, National Heart, Lung, and Blood Institute, National Institute of Allergy and Infectious Diseases, National Institute of Arthritis and Musculoskeletal and Skin Diseases, National Institute of Child Health and Human Development, National Institute of Diabetes and Digestive and Kidney Diseases, National Institute of Handicapped Research, National Institutes of Health, National Institute of Mental Health, National Institute of Neurological and Communicative Disorders and Stroke, National Institute on Aging, National Institute on Alcohol Abuse and Alcoholism, National Institute on Drug Abuse, National Kidney Foundation, National Multiple Sclerosis Society, National Sudden Infant Death Syndrome Foundation, Pharmaceutical Manufacturers Association Commission on Drugs for Rare Diseases, United Cerebral Palsy Association, U.S. Department of Health, Education and Welfare, and the U.S. Surgeon General's Office.

There are many individuals in various Associations, Foundations, and Universities who were also especially helpful. M. Marguerite Donoghue was a valuable resource for information, comment, and support, along with Myrl Weinberg, Len Koch, Joe Isaacs, Dr. Albert Sheffer, John Allegrante, Bob Dresing, Susan Lechtner, Susan Barbe, Corinne Kirchner, Mike Gorman, Dr. Gerald Brackmann, Jan Lipkin, Susan Rappaport, Peter Mathon, Elaine Shelton, Susan Golick, Margaret Gibelman, Dr. Robert Utiger, Dr. George Goldstein, John Donnelly, Dr. Henry Betts, Sean Kennan, Edward Van Ness, Jay Cutler, Nancy Haase, Joyce Waskelo, and Ezell Cox.

Thanks to Alice Fordyce, the Executive Vice President of the Lasker Foundation, always there for encouragement, sound advice, and perspective.

The personal support and friendship of Al and Diane Kaneb and Jack and Rosalind Whitehead gave me the encouragement and resources for such a time-consuming project.

For the beginning research, drafting, and phone calls, I am deeply grateful to Janet Braccio. Her work was continued by Barbara Scherr Trenk, whose outstanding research and writing skills and personal interest were invaluable. Finally, Patricia Bolger did a wonderful job of copyediting.

Undertaking this project took time. I regret the weekends and evenings missed with Connie, Brooke, Trent, and Kyle. It is hoped that the sacrifices of those involved will benefit all of us in our future well-being.

Finally, my father, Lewis William Lierman, whose death from cancer taught me that all statistics have faces and emotions and that, in most instances, the cause of death is lack of research.

Terry L. Lierman
Editor

Building a Healthy America

Medical Research Must Be a National Priority

Saving lives—conquering disease and disability—means alleviating pain and suffering and saving money for the citizens and the country.

—Mary Lasker

What Has the Federal Government Contributed to Research?

The dramatic improvement in the health and longevity of Americans over the past 50 years can be attributed directly to the efforts of our nation's medical research community, an enterprise unparalleled in achievement and unlimited in potential. This unqualified success in both human and economic terms was made possible by the United States government's long-standing commitment to the support of American medical research.

Diseases that once killed or disabled hundreds of thousands of people both here and abroad have been controlled or eradicated. Innovative diagnostic aids, new surgical techniques, and effective drug therapies have eased the management of numerous illnesses and improved the quality of the lives of victims of disease. Promising areas of scientific investigation hold the potential for finally solving many of the medical problems that continue to perplex us. Over the past 50 years, medical research has:

- Virtually eradicated throughout the world such epidemic diseases as smallpox and cholera

- Significantly reduced infant mortality and childhood diseases, such as polio and pertussis

Adapted from *Investing in America's Health: Making the Case for Medical Research*, October 1987, National Health Council, New York, NY.

- Dramatically improved survival rates for patients with cancer, heart disease, and stroke

- Created effective vaccines and drugs to combat serious viral and bacterial diseases, such as hepatitis, rubella, influenza, pneumonia, and meningitis

- Made possible increasingly safe transplantation of vital organs, such as heart, kidneys, and liver

- Developed lifesaving technologies, such as the heart-lung machine, kidney dialysis, cardiac pacemakers, and diagnostic imaging technologies

- Rapidly mobilized research resources in response to new infectious diseases, such as toxic shock syndrome and Legionnaire's disease

- Developed drug therapies for a variety of mental illnesses

- Developed genetic engineering techniques that enable the production of human gene products in the laboratory, resulting in therapies more compatible with the human body

Besides saving and prolonging human lives, America's federal centers for medical research have contributed to an explosion of knowledge that has placed us at the threshold of opportunities not dreamed of 20 years ago. These include:

- The discovery of oncogenes, which can change normal cells into cancer cells and may lead to new methods of cancer control

- The development of monoclonal antibodies, created to attack specific kinds of cancer, which may prove useful in attacking other diseases as well

- The advent of new insulin delivery therapies to help people with diabetes manage their disease and the exploration of implantable insulin-producing cells

- The application of new molecular genetic techniques to the treatment and study of Alzheimer's disease and our understanding of the aging process

What Are the Economic Gains of Investing in Medical Research?

The economic returns of America's investment in medical research are impressive. Studies indicate that the rate of return on every $1 invested in medical research is as high as $13. These dollar amounts reflect savings from reductions in absenteeism, lost productivity, and direct and indirect medical expenses. Over $10 was returned for every $1 invested in the research, development, and application of the measles vaccine, a nearly $4.5 billion return. Medical research annually contributes an estimated $40 billion to our economy, which is used in nonhealth fields. The introduction of lithium treatment for manic-depressive illness has saved $6.5 billion, far exceeding the total federal investment in medical research at the National Institute of Mental Health

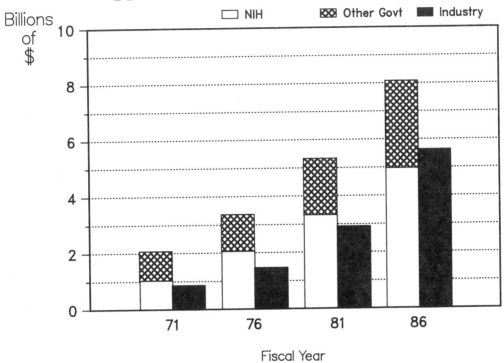

NIH, Other Government and Industry Support of Health R&D, FY 1971–1986

Source: NIH 1982 and 1986 Data Books. Other Government includes federal, state, and local

(NIMH) within the Alcohol, Drug Abuse, and Mental Health Administration (ADAMHA).

What Is the Cost of Inadequate Funding?

The continuing need to address health problems can be expressed in economic terms as well as in human terms. For example, U.S. health care spending in 1985, the latest year for which complete figures are available, totalled $456.4 billion, consuming 10.8 percent of our Gross National Product (GNP). Yet the federal government's expenditure on medical research, which can contribute significantly to reducing health care costs, was only 1.2 percent of that figure (down from nearly 3 percent of total health care spending 20 years ago). The annual per capita expenditure in the United States for health care is approximately $2,000; the per capita expenditure on health research is only about $25.

Disease threatens the health and well-being of both our citizens and our economy, and there is the additional threat posed by foreign competitors to our preeminence in research. Japan and West Germany have made strong national commitments to investing in research and high technology. In 1985, each of these countries spent about 2.6 percent of their GNP on civilian research and development expenditures; the current United States expenditure level is only 1.8 percent. In the 1980s, over 45 percent of all U.S. patents granted in the field of drugs and medicine have been awarded to foreign inventors.

Uncertainty is growing about the ability of America's medical research enterprise to remain vital and strong without a heightened federal commitment to ensure it. Popular support for federal funding of medical research is strong. An overwhelming number of Americans believe that "government funds for basic research should be increased by a sizeable amount—even in this era of tight federal budgets and soaring deficits," according to a December 1983 Louis Harris poll.

High federal deficits have made medical research an easy target for the Administration's budget axe, yet research spending on defense programs, which have a demonstrably lower rate of return on investment, has skyrocketed. These efforts to curtail federal spending on medical research are producing an unstable environment within the medical research community. One negative impact is the loss of promising young scientific investigators from their chosen medical field. This is critical because the continued integrity of the nation's medical research enterprise will depend heavily on the availability of a pool of talented researchers, which is now in serious jeopardy.

Why Should the Federal Government Be the Prime Sponsor of Medical Research?

The most appropriate underwriter of medical research in this country has been and must continue to be the federal government. Although its private sector partners in discovery—business, academia, and voluntary health organizations—have made invaluable contributions to the battle against death and disease, a simple fact remains: medical research, like many other forms of basic research, is a high-risk enterprise that demands a large-scale societal commitment best led by our federal government.

America's medical researchers have achieved their impressive track record because of a central, commonly shared principle: although it may be unpredictable and time-consuming, exploring the frontiers of science will yield the most fruitful results if research is concentrated foremost on the fundamental exploration of basic life processes.

The one source able to provide adequate human and financial resources to undertake this effort remains the federal centers for medical research. In recent years, however, there has been a decline in administration support for what had become a traditional federal responsibility—funding medical research. Increased funding is urgently needed to:

• Attract and continually replenish an adequate corps of highly trained and productive scientific investigators

- Rehabilitate, renovate, or replace deteriorating research facilities and outmoded technology and equipment

- Expand promising fields of scientific inquiry to address America's urgent, growing health needs

- Improve the communication of important research findings not only to the scientific community but also to medical practitioners and the ultimate consumer—the general public

The health needs of America have become more pressing, while promising avenues for discovery go unexplored and our position of dominance in the world research community is eroding. The cornerstone of American medical research has been the dedication of ample federal support. Adequate resources are the lifeline of medical research, and a strong medical research enterprise is ultimately the lifeline of America.

The Role of the Federal Government in Health

*If you are looking about for examples
of things that government can do, and
do beautifully well, rest your eyes on
the NIH. The existence of this
institution in its present form owes
much to the political leaders in and
out of Congress, whose wisdom and
statecraft put it in place.*

— *Lewis Thomas, M.D.*
Lasker Foundation Awards, 1986

What Is the Department of Health and Human Services?

The Department of Health and Human Services (DHHS) is a cabinet-level department
of the federal government's executive branch. The DHHS touches the lives of more
Americans than any other federal agency. At one time or another, every citizen of the
United States benefits from at least one of the department's programs, which range
from prenatal care to social security.

There are four major divisions within the DHHS:

1. Public Health Service

2. Office of Human Development Services

3. Health Care Financing Administration

4. Social Security Administration

The Public Health Service (PHS) promotes the protection and advancement of the
nation's health through research, service, and prevention programs. The Office of
Human Development Services provides leadership and direction to human services
programs for children, the elderly, families, Native Americans, people living in rural

Department of Health and Human Services

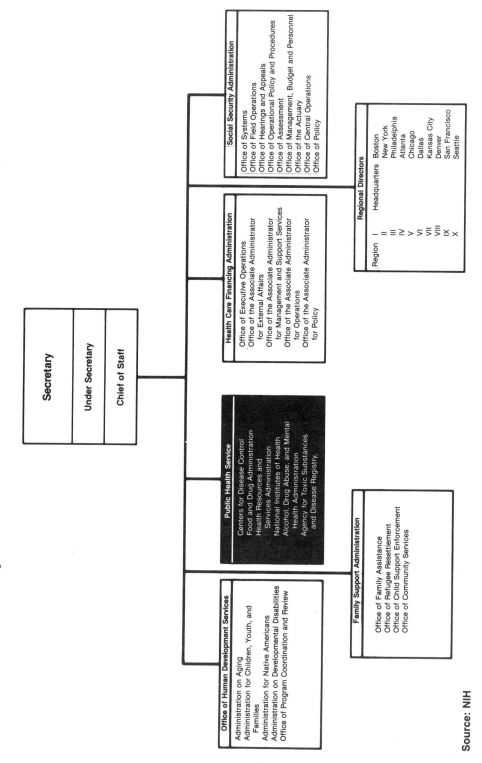

Source: NIH

areas, handicapped people, and public assistance recipients. The Health Care Financing Administration (HCFA) oversees the Medicare and Medicaid programs.

The Social Security Administration administers a national program of contributory social insurance; employees, employers, and the self-employed make contributions that are pooled in special trust funds. When earnings stop or are reduced because the worker retires, dies, or becomes disabled, monthly cash benefits are paid to replace some of the earnings the family has lost.

What Is the Public Health Service?

The PHS is responsible for the nation's health. The Assistant Secretary for Health and the Surgeon General are responsible for the programs of the PHS, which is comprised of six major subdivisions:

1. National Institutes of Health (NIH)

2. Alcohol, Drug Abuse, and Mental Health Administration (ADAMHA)

3. Centers for Disease Control (CDC)

4. Food and Drug Administration (FDA)

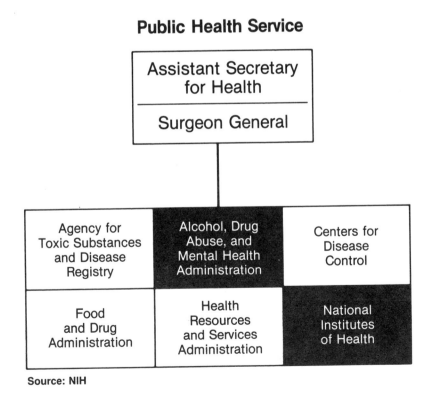

Public Health Service

Assistant Secretary for Health
Surgeon General

Agency for Toxic Substances and Disease Registry	Alcohol, Drug Abuse, and Mental Health Administration	Centers for Disease Control
Food and Drug Administration	Health Resources and Services Administration	National Institutes of Health

Source: NIH

5. Health Resources and Services Administration (HRSA)

6. Agency for Toxic Substances and Disease Registry

The Office of the Assistant Secretary for Health consists of two major operating centers:

1. The National Center for Health Statistics collects, analyzes, and disseminates statistics on vital events and health activities to reflect health status, health needs, and health resources.

2. The National Center for Health Services Research plans, develops, and administers a program of health services research, demonstrations, evaluations, and research training.

The Surgeon General is the highest ranking officer in the Commissioned Corps. This office supports the Assistant Secretary for Health in providing leadership and direction for the Public Health Service.

The NIH is the principal medical research agency in the federal government; with ADAMHA, it promotes strategies for solving health problems, including issues associated with the use and abuse of alcohol and drugs and mental health problems.

The Centers for Disease Control (CDC) is the federal agency that provides leadership and direction in the prevention and control of diseases and other medical conditions.

The Food and Drug Administration (FDA) works to protect the health of the nation against impure and unsafe foods, drugs and cosmetics, and medical devices.

The Health Resources and Services Administration (HRSA) provides leadership and direction to programs and activities designed to improve health services and to develop health care and maintenance systems that are adequately financed, comprehensive, interrelated, and responsive to the needs of individuals and families in all levels of society.

The Agency for Toxic Substances and Disease Registry directs programs and activities designed to protect both the public health and worker safety from the adverse health effects of hazardous substances in storage sites or released in fires, explosions, or transportation accidents.

What Are the National Institutes of Health?

The mission of the NIH is to improve the health of the nation by increasing understanding of human health, disability, and disease, advancing knowledge about the health effects of the environment, and developing and improving methods of preventing, detecting, diagnosing, and treating disease.

NIH accomplishes this mission through:

- Support of medical research in universities, hospitals, and research institutions in this country and abroad

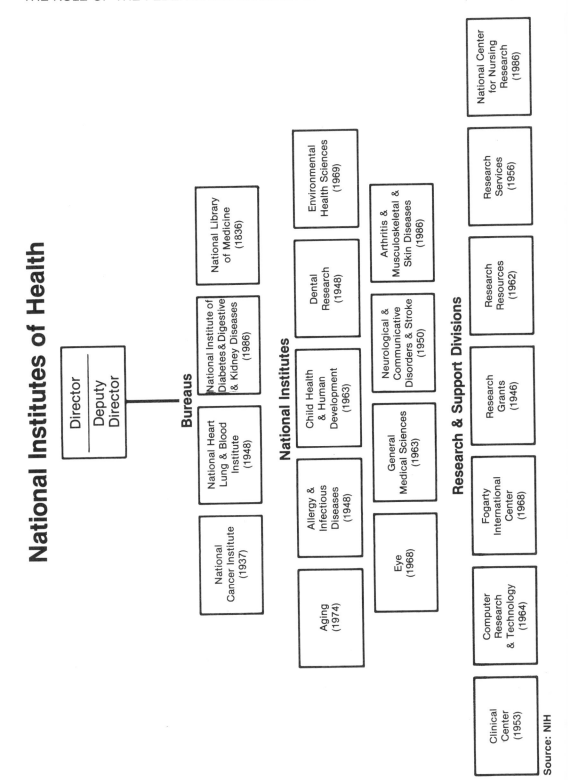

National Institutes of Health

Bureaus

Director
Deputy Director

- National Cancer Institute (1937)
- National Heart Lung & Blood Institute (1948)
- National Institute of Diabetes & Digestive & Kidney Diseases (1986)
- National Library of Medicine (1836)

National Institutes

- Aging (1974)
- Allergy & Infectious Diseases (1948)
- Child Health & Human Development (1963)
- Dental Research (1948)
- Environmental Health Sciences (1969)
- Eye (1968)
- General Medical Sciences (1963)
- Neurological & Communicative Disorders & Stroke (1950)
- Arthritis & Musculoskeletal & Skin Diseases (1986)

Research & Support Divisions

- Clinical Center (1953)
- Computer Research & Technology (1964)
- Fogarty International Center (1968)
- Research Grants (1946)
- Research Resources (1962)
- Research Services (1956)
- National Center for Nursing Research (1986)

Source: NIH

- Conduct of medical research in its own laboratories and clinics

- Support of training for promising young researchers

- Development and maintenance of research resources

- Identification of research advances that have significant potential for clinical application and transfer of these advances to the health care system

- Promotion of effective ways to communicate biomedical information to scientists, health practitioners, and the public

Organizational Structure

To carry out its mission and legislative mandates, the NIH is organized into an Office of the Director, the National Library of Medicine, and the following institutes:

- National Cancer Institute

- National Eye Institute

- National Heart, Lung, and Blood Institute

- National Institute on Aging

- National Institute of Allergy and Infectious Diseases

- National Institute of Arthritis and Musculoskeletal and Skin Diseases

- National Institute of Child Health and Human Development

- National Institute of Dental Research

- National Institute of Diabetes and Digestive and Kidney Diseases

- National Institute of Environmental Health Sciences

- National Institute of General Medical Sciences

- National Institute of Neurological and Communicative Disorders and Stroke

- National Center for Nursing Research

The NIH also includes the Warren Grant Magnuson Clinical Center, a combined 500-bed research hospital and laboratory complex, and the Fogarty International Center, which fosters international biomedical research collaboration. All of the 13 NIH Institutes, the Division of Research Resources, the Fogarty Center, and the National Library of Medicine have individual congressional appropriations. In total, the NIH receives 16 separate appropriations each year.

NIH is staffed by 12,000 employees, including more than 3,200 scientists (about 1,250 with M.D.s and 1,800 with Ph.D.s). Its budget, which exceeds $6 billion, supports far more than the buildings, laboratories, and people on the Bethesda, Maryland, campus. More than 80 percent of the NIH budget funds the projects of nearly 20,000 scientists in 1,300 universities, medical schools, hospitals, and other research

Getting a NIH grant

```
Initiates                                                              Manages
research idea                                                          fund
and prepares
application

                              Investigator

                        National Institutes Of Health

Submits                                                               Investigator
application                                                          conducts
                                                                     research

NIH division of    Peer review    Institute        Advisory board    Institute makes
research grants    group          evaluates        recommends        funding
assigns to study   evaluates for  program          action            selections and
section and one of scientific     relevance and                      issues grant
11 institutes      merit          need                                awards
```

Source: National Institutes Of Health

Source: The Sacramento Bee, September 15–October 3, 1985

institutions throughout the United States and abroad. NIH-supported scientists pursue their own scientific ideas through extramural research grants. These and other programs, including the training of young scientists, have proven to be powerful mechanisms for fostering scientific discovery.

A Century of Science for Health

The year 1987 marks 100 years of biomedical research at NIH or, as the centennial theme states, "A Century of Science for Health." The NIH began as the Hygienic Laboratory, a one-room facility in the Marine Health Service Hospital on Staten Island. The sole researcher was Dr. Joseph Kinyoun, a physician and bacteriologist who had worked in the laboratories of Louis Pasteur and Robert Koch. The Hygienic Laboratory moved to Washington in 1891, and the Ransdell Act of 1930 designated the Hygienic Laboratory as the National Institute of Health. The cornerstone for the first building at the Bethesda campus was laid June 30, 1938. Since then, the NIH has grown to over 40 buildings encompassing 311 acres.

The research programs of the NIH have generated discoveries that have led to lower death rates from heart disease, cancer, stroke, and respiratory distress syndrome of the newborn. Research scientists who are supported by NIH or who work in its laboratories in Bethesda and elsewhere have developed improved vaccines for influenza, pneumococcal pneumonia, rubella, rabies, hepatitis, and other infectious diseases that once caused handicapping illness and death.

What Is the Alcohol, Drug Abuse, and Mental Health Administration?

ADAMHA was established by Congress in 1974 to administer and coordinate national programs to improve understanding and prevention of alcohol and drug abuse and mental health disorders. ADAMHA has three institutes: the National Institute on Al-

The National Institutes of Health (NIH)

Mission

NIH has the principal responsibility within the federal government for improving the health of the nation through the conduct and support of research and research training. The objective is to sustain the present quality and level of biomedical research capabilities nationally, assuring progress across a broad range of activities. NIH:

- Stimulates the development of an ever expanding scientific base

- Assesses new therapeutic techniques and facilitates their transfer into health practice

- Provides the knowledge and scientific base for the development and growth of whole new areas of technology

- Ensures the continuing availability of a pool of skilled investigators

NIH does not provide health services other than therapeutic measures and care incidental to research and has no regulatory responsibilities other than recommending standards for the use of animal and human subjects in federally supported health research and in the conduct of recombinant DNA research.

Organization and Programs

Brief descriptions of the divisions of the NIH follow, along with the telephone number of the Information Office.

- **The National Cancer Institute** conducts and supports research relating to the cause, prevention, and treatment of cancer and conducts a program in cancer control embracing cancer detection and diagnosis, therapy, rehabilitation, and education. (301) 496–6631

- **The National Eye Institute** conducts and supports research to gain new knowledge and understanding of the eye and visual system, the pathology of visual disorders, and scientific information essential to progress against the major causes of blindness and visual disability. (301) 496–5248

- **The National Heart, Lung, and Blood Institute** conducts and supports a national program in research on diseases of the heart, blood vessels, lung, and blood and in the management of blood resources. The program encompasses the full spectrum of basic laboratory research, clinical investigation, validation of promising findings through clinical trials, and the translation of research findings as well as the training and career development of investigators. (301) 496–4236

- **The National Institute of Allergy and Infectious Diseases** conducts and supports broadly based research and research training on the causes, characterization, prevention, control, and treatment of a wide variety of diseases believed to be caused by infectious agents or disorders in the body's immune mechanisms. (301) 496–5717

- **The National Institute of Arthritis and Musculoskeletal and Skin Diseases** conducts, fosters, and supports basic and clinical research into the causes, prevention, diagnosis, and treatment of arthritis, musculoskeletal disorders, and skin diseases. (301) 496–8188

- **The National Institute of Child Health and Human Development** conducts and supports research on the reproductive, developmental, and behavioral processes that determine the health of children, adults, families, and populations. (301) 496–5133

- **The National Institute of Dental Research** is responsible for research into the causes, prevention, diagnosis, and treatment of oral and dental diseases. It conducts and supports clinical and laboratory research directed toward the eradication of tooth decay and a broad array of oral–facial disorders. (301) 496–4261

- **The National Institute of Diabetes and Digestive and Kidney Diseases** conducts and supports basic and clinical research into the causes, prevention, diagnosis, and treatment of diabetes mellitus, endocrine and metabolic diseases, digestive diseases and nutritional disorders, and kidney, urologic, and hematologic diseases. (301) 496–3583

- **The National Institute of Environmental Health Sciences** investigates the effects of chemical, physical, and biologic environmental agents on human health. Its goal is to provide the scientific information base, advanced methodology, and trained manpower to improve the understanding of the impact of environmental factors on human health. (919) 541–3345

- **The National Institute of General Medical Sciences** supports research and research training in the sciences basic to medicine. It works to gain increased knowledge in the fundamental life sciences and to support research in such fields as genetics, cell biology, molecular biology, and pharmacology because progress in these areas is essential to success against the various diseases represented by the other NIH institutes. (301) 496–7301

- **The National Institute of Neurological and Communicative Disorders and Stroke** studies a wide range of disorders of the nervous system, the neuromuscular apparatus, the ear, human communication, and the special senses of taste, smell, touch, and pain. (301) 496–5924

- **The National Institute on Aging** is responsible for biomedical behavioral, and social research on the aging process, diseases, and other special problems and needs of the aged. (301) 496–1752

- **The National Center for Nursing Research** conducts and supports basic and clinical nursing research, training, and other programs in patient care research and information dissemination. (301) 496–8230

- **The John E. Fogarty International Center for Advanced Education in the Health Sciences** fosters and coordinates NIH international cooperation in the life sciences, brings internationally known scientists to the NIH campus, supports senior scientists between the United States and other countries under bilateral agreements, and serves as a focal point for foreign visitors to the NIH. (301) 496–2075

- **The Division of Computer Research and Technology** is responsible for incorporating modern computer technology into NIH biomedical research and administrative procedures. It also serves as a scientific and technologic resource for other federal agencies with biomedical and computing needs. (301) 496–6203

- **The Warren G. Magnuson Clinical Center** is a combined 540-bed research hospital and laboratory complex that provides high-quality patient care necessary to conduct research and is designed so that bench scientists in some 1,100 laboratories can work together with clinicians caring for patients and collaborate closely on mutual research problems. Unlike most hospitals, the Clinical Center does not offer general diagnostic, emergency, and treatment services. Patients are selected solely because they have an illness that is being studied under a formal research protocol by one or more of the Institutes. Recently completed is a 13-story Ambulatory Care Research Facility to provide space for the hospital's expanding outpatient research program. (301) 496–2563

- **The Division of Research Grants** is the nerve center for the NIH grants programs. It administers grant applications, provides for their scientific review, and helps formulate grant and award policies and procedures. (301) 496–7441

- **The Division of Research Resources** administers programs aimed at developing and ensuring the availability of resources essential to the effective conduct of health research. It helps institutions establish and operate general clinical research centers, supports highly sophisticated resources, such as computer centers, primate research centers, and laboratory animal facilities, makes awards to minority individuals and institutions to engage in biomedical research, and provides support through formula grants to enhance the efficiency and effectiveness of biomedical and behavioral research at institutions receiving PHS grant support. (301) 496–5545

- **The Division of Research Services** provides a variety of centralized services for NIH scientists, such as environmental health and safety services, provision of animals needed for research, biomedical engineering and instrumentation services, medical library and translating services, and medical illustration, design graphics, and photographic services. (301) 496–5795

- **The National Library of Medicine** is the world's most complete reference center devoted to a single subject, with a collection including 2.5 million items. The Library has pioneered the use of such technology as automated information retrieval, computer-assisted publishing, and communications satellites to make its resources available to scientists and practitioners all across the nation. In addition, its Lister Hill Center for Biomedical Communications conducts research in electronic document storage, retrieval, and dissemination systems and in the development of computerized knowledge base systems derived from the scientific literature and organized for easy access by the practicing physician. (301) 496–6308

cohol Abuse and Alcoholism (NIAAA), the National Institute on Drug Abuse (NIDA), and the National Institute of Mental Health (NIMH). The chief mission of these institutes is to advance scientific knowledge through the conduct and support of basic and applied scientific research.

The Office of the Administrator coordinates the Institutes' activities.

National Institute on Alcohol Abuse and Alcoholism

NIAAA conducts and supports a wide range of studies on the causes, consequences, and treatment of alcohol abuse and alcoholism and alcohol-related medical disorders. The Institute also seeks ways to prevent these problems and ways to intervene early, especially with highly vulnerable populations, such as youth, children of alcoholics, and women of childbearing age.

The recently established Laboratory of Clinical Studies at the NIH includes inpatient and outpatient programs designed to study health problems associated with alcohol abuse and alcoholism, including defining the pathology of alcoholism and developing appropriate pharmacologic and related diagnostic, treatment, and prevention approaches.

National Institute on Drug Abuse

NIDA supports research in scientific centers around the country on the complex biologic, behavioral, and epidemiologic factors involved in drug abuse. Basic research is conducted on the mechanisms of drug action in brain and body and on the effects of specific drugs, including heroin and other narcotics, marijuana, cocaine, stimulants, sedatives and hypnotics, PCP, LSD, and others. NIDA also supports research on the addictive properties of nicotine.

The Institute sponsors national surveys to determine changing patterns of illicit drug use throughout the country and identify the characteristics of people who use drugs. NIDA-supported research scientists are seeking more effective approaches to treating and preventing drug abuse. New research findings relevant to treatment are rapidly and widely disseminated to physicians and other practitioners who provide care to drug abusers.

National Institute of Mental Health

NIMH supports a wide range of scientific studies in universities, hospitals, and other research centers to advance knowledge of the biologic, genetic, and environmental bases for behavior and effective new ways to treat and prevent mental illness. Other mental health research is aimed at better understanding of family processes, the causes of stress in people's lives, and their coping mechanisms. Some research aims at developing new therapies and assessing the efficacy and safety of treatment methods being used.

NIMH conducts and supports epidemiology research to collect national data on the incidence and prevalence of mental illnesses. The studies indicate the mental health status of various segments of the United States population and assess their risk for mental and emotional disorders. In research on how to prevent these disorders, NIMH supports studies of ways to promote healthy behaviors and coping skills, such as the most effective ways to help people who have undergone a life crisis. A special focus of the Institute's prevention studies is people considered at risk for mental and emotional problems, including children of parents who are mentally ill, substance abusers, or separated or divorced.

Source

National Institutes of Health

How Congress Works for Health

Health is the first wealth of the nation.

— *Senator Warren Magnuson*

What Is the Role of Congressional Committees in the Legislative Process?

January 6, 1987, was the first day of the 100th Congress of the United States. This year also marks the 200th anniversary of the Constitution and the form of government we know today. The adoption of the Constitution centralized many rights and responsibilities of the federal government, and the congressional process has remained essentially the same since that time.

Today, as it was 200 years ago, each Congress consists of two sessions, with each session running 1 year. At the end of each Congress, all 435 seats of the House of Representatives and one third of the 100 seats of the United States Senate must be decided by election.

At the beginning of each Congress, committee chairmen are appointed or reappointed, and members are assigned to the committees. There are 16 major committees in the Senate and 22 in the House of Representatives. The committee structure in Congress is absolute, emphasizing the critical importance of committee assignments. The Congress of the United States conducts its daily business within the committee system.

In the 99th Congress, more than 11,500 bills and resolutions were introduced. With very few exceptions, these bills either originated in committees or were referred to a committee for action. Over 700 of these bills were related to health.

Why Are Committees Important?

Committees are the heart of the legislative process for both authorization and appropriations. They have existed in the Senate and the House since 1789 and have allowed for a division of work and orderly consideration of legislation. The size of the Senate (100 members) and the House (435 voting members) makes it difficult for all members to consider each piece of legislation. Consequently, each chamber has established its own committees to study and consider legislation. In turn, committees have established subcommittees to allow even further division of work. The Senate and House have similar committee titles and structure.

Which Committees Have the Most Impact on Health Programs?

Eight committees have the most impact on health legislation.

Authorization Committees

- Senate Committee on Finance
  Subcommittee on Health
- House Committee on Ways and Means
- Senate Committee on Labor and Human Resources
- House Committee on Energy and Commerce
  Subcommittee on Health and the Environment

Appropriations Committees

- Senate Committee on Appropriations
  Subcommittee on Labor, Health and Human Services, Education and Related Agencies
- House Committee on Appropriations
  Subcommittee on Labor, Health and Human Services, Education and Related Agencies

Congressional Budget Committees

- Senate Committee on the Budget
- House Committee on the Budget

Authorization Committees

These committees create laws that establish in statute specific ideas and particular programs, including their mission, goals, and often how to implement objectives. Authorizing legislation sets levels of spending that are usually not exceeded by the appropriations committees. Some health programs have an open-ended authorization, which means that there is no maximum on the amount of money that can be appropriated for a program.

Authorizing responsibility for most health programs is divided among four congressional committees. In the House of Representatives, authorizing jurisdiction generally is related to the source of funding. For example, the House Committee on Ways and Means is responsible for programs funded from revenues raised through payroll taxes, such as Medicare. The House Committee on Energy and Commerce is responsible for health care programs funded through general revenues, such as the block grants, Medicaid, and biomedical research. In the Senate, jurisdiction is divided by authorizing statute. The Senate Committee on Finance, for example, handles the Social Security Act, including Medicare, Medicaid, and Maternal and Child Health. The Senate Committee on Labor and Human Resources authorizes spending programs covered by the Public Health Service Act and other laws covering discretionary health programs. Discretionary health programs are funded at the discretion of Congress, for example, research, training, and prevention programs and community health centers. Nondiscretionary programs or entitlement programs are those that, by law, must be funded, such as Medicaid and Medicare.

Appropriations Committees

In order to be funded, a program must pass through the appropriations process. These committees generally act after a program is authorized. The Committee on Appropriations determines how a program will be funded and at what level. The only restriction is the authorized ceiling or maximum. Authorization of a program does not guarantee that it will be funded.

Congressional Budget Committees

The budget committees review proposed broad levels of expenditures so that Congress as a whole knows how much money will be spent if all bills are enacted and all taxes collected. This determines what the federal deficit — or surplus — will be. The committee then sets targets or ceilings within which the authorization and appropriations committees must act.

How Are Committee Appointments Made?

Membership ratios on committees between the majority and minority parties are determined at the beginning of each Congress and reflect the ratio that exists for the entire membership of each chamber as well as the political judgment of the majority party. Members are assigned to committees by caucus of the respective parties, and these assignments are confirmed by a floor vote. The chairman is usually the committee member of the majority party with the most years of service in Congress. The most senior member of the minority party is usually designated ranking minority member.

Congressional Committees on Health

House Committee on Ways and Means
Subcommittee on Health

Chairman: Fortney (Pete) Stark (D-California)
Rep. Brian J. Donnelly (D-Massachusetts)
Rep. J.J. Pickle (D-Texas)
Rep. Beryl Anthony (D-Arkansas)
Rep. Sander M. Levin (D-Michigan)
Rep. Jim Moody (D-Wisconsin)
Rep. Willis D. Gradison (R-Ohio)
Rep. Hal Daub (R-Nebraska)
Rep. Judd Gregg (R-New Hampshire)
Rep. Rod Chandler (R-Washington)

House Committee on Appropriations
Subcommittee on Labor, Health and Human Services,
Education and Related Agencies

Chairman: William Natcher (D-Kentucky)
Rep. Neal Smith (D-Iowa)
Rep. David Obey (D-Wisconsin)
Rep. Edward Roybal (D-California)
Rep. Louis Stokes (D-Ohio)
Rep. Joseph Early (D-Massachusetts)
Rep. Bernard Dwyer (D-New Jersey)
Rep. Steny Hoyer (D-Maryland)
Rep. Silvio Conte (R-Massachusetts)
Rep. Carl Pursell (R-Michigan)
Rep. John Edward Porter (R-Illinois)
Rep. C.W. Bill Young (R-Florida)
Rep. Vin Weber (R-Minnesota)

House Committee on Energy and Commerce
Subcommittee on Health and the Environment

Chairman: Henry Waxman (D-California)
Rep. James Scheuer (D-New York)
Rep. Doug Walgren (D-Pennsylvania)

Rep. Ron Wyden (D-Oregon)
Rep. Gerry Sikorski (D-Minnesota)
Rep. Jim Bates (D-California)
Rep. Terry Bruce (D-Illinois)
Rep. Mickey Leland (D-Texas)
Rep. Cardiss Collins (D-Illinois)
Rep. Ralph M. Hall (D-Texas)
Rep. Wayne Dowdy (D-Mississippi)
Rep. John Dingell (D-Michigan) (Ex officio)
Rep. Edward Madigan (R-Illinois)
Rep. William Dannemeyer (R-California)
Rep. Bob Whittaker (R-Kansas)
Rep. Thomas J. Tauke (R-Iowa)
Rep. Dan Coats (R-Indiana)
Rep. Thomas Bliley (R-Virginia)
Rep. Jack Fields (R-Texas)
Rep. Norman Lent (R-New York)

Senate Committee on Appropriations
Subcommittee on Labor, Health and Human Services, Education and Related Agencies

Chairman: Lawton Chiles (D-Florida)
Sen. Robert Byrd (D-West Virginia)
Sen. William Proxmire (D-Wisconsin)
Sen. Ernest Hollings (D-South Carolina)
Sen. Quentin Burdick (D-North Dakota)
Sen. Daniel Inouye (D-Hawaii)
Sen. Tom Harkin (D-Iowa)
Sen. Dale Bumpers (D-Arkansas)
Sen. Lowell P. Weicker (R-Connecticut)
Sen. Mark Hatfield (R-Oregon)
Sen. Ted Stevens (D-Alaska)
Sen. Warren Rudman (R-New Hampshire)
Sen. Arlen Specter (D-Pennsylvania)
Sen. James McClure (R-Idaho)
Sen. Pete Domenici (R-New Mexico)

Senate Committee on Finance
Subcommittee on Health

Chairman: George Mitchell (D-Maine)
Sen. Lloyd Bentsen (D-Texas)
Sen. Max Baucus (D-Montana)

Sen. Bill Bradley (D-New Jersey)
Sen. David Pryor (D-Arkansas)
Sen. Donald Riegle (D-Michigan)
Sen. John Rockefeller (D-West Virginia)
Sen. Dave Durenberger (R-Minnesota)
Sen. Bob Packwood (R-Oregon)
Sen. Bob Dole (R-Kansas)
Sen. John Chafee (R-Rhode Island)
Sen. John Heinz (R-Pennsylvania)

Senate Committee on Labor and Human Resources

Chairman: Edward Kennedy (D-Massachusetts)
Sen. Claiborne Pell (D-Rhode Island)
Sen. Howard Metzenbaum (D-Ohio)
Sen. Spark Matsunaga (D-Hawaii)
Sen. Christopher Dodd (D-Connecticut)
Sen. Paul Simon (D-Illinois)
Sen. Tom Harkin (D-Iowa)
Sen. Brock Adams (D-Washington)
Sen. Barbara Mikulski (D-Maryland)
Sen. Orrin Hatch (R-Utah)
Sen. Robert Stafford (R-Vermont)
Sen. Dan Quayle (D-Indiana)
Sen. Strom Thurmond (R-South Carolina)
Sen. Lowell Weicker (R-Connecticut)
Sen. Thad Cochran (R-Mississippi)
Sen. Gordon Humphrey (R-New Hampshire)

The full committee then determines subcommittee membership, maintaining the same majority/minority ratios. In general, senators may serve on two major committees and as many as eight subcommittees. In the House, a representative usually serves on one or two committees.

Subcommittees and committees are responsible to their parent bodies, although they have substantial independence and autonomy. The chairman of a committee or subcommittee is a dominant figure in the legislative process because he or she can determine which issues are considered and the pace at which the legislative process moves. Most bills referred to a committee are not acted on, and only a few become law, since many are duplicative or do not have sufficient support.

What Role Does Committee Staff Play?

Because of the magnitude of issues that concern Congress and the impossible task of a senator or representative to be fully informed on all issues, Congress hires professional staff to assist committees with their activities. In 1969, there were five professionals to staff the six major health committees. By 1987, this number had increased to approximately 70 because Congress has attempted to develop its own research capabilities rather than rely entirely on the executive branch.

A participant in the legislative process should be cognizant of the important role the committee staff and a member's personal staff play. Their advice and counsel are sought and respected by senators and representatives, although the extent to which members of Congress depend on staff support varies greatly. Staff are generally receptive to information and ideas. They are there to serve the committee and its members. A sympathetic ear from staff, given the right issue and the member's priorities, can greatly enhance the legislation's outlook and assist the members to do their jobs.

How Is a Bill Authorized and Funded?

There are four basic forms in which a proposal or idea may be introduced. The most common is a bill, which is numbered separately for the Senate and the House in order of introduction during a session of Congress. Senate bills are designated with the letter S. for Senate, and House bills with the letters H.R. for House of Representatives.

The three other forms are joint resolutions, concurrent resolutions, and simple resolutions. Joint resolutions may originate in either the Senate or the House (S.J. Res. or H.J. Res. followed by a sequential number). Little difference exists between a bill and a joint resolution. The terms can be used interchangeably.

Concurrent resolutions (S. Con. Res. or H. Con. Res. followed by a sequential number) are used for matters that affect the operations of both the Senate and the House. This would include a concurrent resolution of the budget directing committees to take certain actions. In addition, they can express the sense of Congress on facts, principles, and opinions. Concurrent resolutions are not legislative in character.

Simple resolutions (S. Res. or H. Res. followed by a sequential number) generally concern matters that affect only the operations of either the Senate or the House. They are considered only by their respective bodies.

Introduction and Referral

The first step in the legislative process for authorization bills is the introduction of the bill and its referral to an appropriate committee. In the Senate, a member asks for recognition by the presiding officer to introduce a bill and will often include floor remarks on the nature of the bill. In the House, a member presents the bill to the Clerk of the House or places it in a box near the Speaker's platform called the "hopper." It is common for a senator and representative to sponsor identical bills, each introducing his or her version simultaneously in his or her respective chamber.

After assigning the bill an appropriate number, the presiding officer refers it to the appropriate standing committees. The committee then refers the bill to one of its subcommittees unless the chairman decides to have the full committee act on the proposal. When a bill involves more than one committee, it may be jointly referred or successively referred to more than one committee. Successive referral, the most common form, allows one committee to take action first. It then refers the bill to the second committee. An example of joint referral in the 98th Congress was the 1984 Deficit Reduction Act. This proposed legislation was jointly referred to the House Committee on Energy and Commerce and the Committee on Ways and Means.

Senators or representatives who are interested in actively promoting their legislation often will seek cosponsors. This allows other legislators to jointly introduce the bill, indicating their support for it. Bipartisan sponsorship can be very important, as can endorsement by members of the committee to which the bill will be referred. There is no limit on the number of cosponsors that can be added to a House or Senate bill or resolution.

Hearings

When a committee or subcommittee decides to act on a legislative proposal, generally hearings are conducted. These hearings provide the opportunity for the executive branch, interested groups, and individuals to present their views on the legislative topic. Transcripts of hearings are recorded and printed for committee and public use.

Depending on the nature of a bill, hearings may be conducted for a few hours or for several days or weeks. Sometimes, but not often, the chairman of the committee or subcommittee will limit the type and number of individuals and organizations that may testify. This is done either to expedite the committee's deliberations or to create a particular atmosphere at the hearing. It is becoming more common for committees and subcommittees to hold educational hearings to inform members on current issues.

It is during this step that the affected federal agencies and the General Accounting Office may be asked for written comments and views on the bill under consideration.

How a House-proposed Bill Travels Through the Congressional Maze

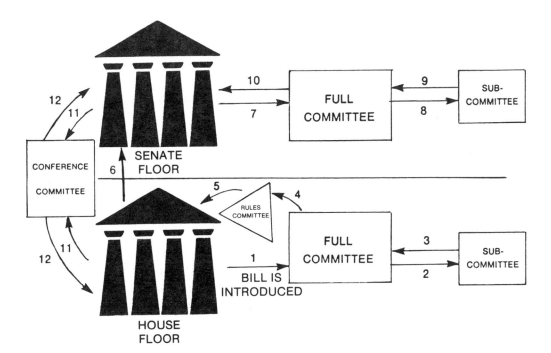

Oversight

In addition to legislative functions, committees and subcommittees have the power to conduct oversight hearings. Both Senate and House rules give committees jurisdiction to carry out oversight responsibilities, and some subcommittees are created exclusively for this role. The purpose of oversight is to analyze, appraise, and evaluate both the execution and effectiveness of laws administered by the executive branch and to determine if there are areas in which additional legislation is necessary or desirable.

Recently, various health committees conducted oversight hearings on the Prospective Payment System for Medicare, Peer Review Organizations, graduate medical education, and intermediate care facilities for the mentally retarded.

Oversight will continue to play an important role in the development of health policy by increasing the accountability of both the federal government and the private sector.

Mark-Up

Upon completion of hearings, the committee or subcommittee will proceed to mark-up the bill or bills it has considered. The term "marking-up" means changing or amending and is coined from the line-by-line review given a bill by the committee. During this step of the process, a member may offer amendments. As a rule, informal votes are taken on each change or amendment in order to obtain a consensus.

When the subcommittee has completed action, the bill is reported out or ordered reported to the full committee. If the bill has been amended substantially during mark-up, the subcommittee may redraft it as a clean bill, incorporating all amendments in new bill language. The clean bill is then reintroduced, assigned a new number, and referred to the full committee. This allows further deliberations on a document that is simplified and unencumbered with numerous amendments.

Seldom does a full committee take the time to deliberate the issues or policies in the depth that the subcommittee has. Discussion is more general, and although amendments may be offered, they are usually fewer than those considered in subcommittee. As mentioned earlier, because of the number and scope of issues, committees generally rely on and accept the conclusions of the subcommittee. There are exceptions to this generalization, however; for example, the Senate Committee on Finance considers Medicare–Medicaid legislation at the full committee level, and the Senate Committee on Labor and Human Resources has no health subcommittee.

When the committee completes its deliberations, the bill is again reported out or ordered reported — this time to the Senate or House floor for a vote. Accompanying the bill is a bill report. These reports, numbered sequentially as reported to the Senate or House (e.g., S. Report 100-1, 100-2, 100-3), may include an analysis of the legislative language, a history of the bill, a review of existing legislation, and a statement of the committee's reasons or intent for passing on the bill. Minority views or dissenting opinions may also become part of the report.

After a bill becomes law, there may be confusion or ambiguity in the actual legislative language. When this occurs, the committee report may be useful to determine the congressional intent of the bill. For example, when the executive branch writes regulations and the courts rule on legislation, they will often rely on this background if the law itself is not clear.

Increasingly over the last few years, mark-up has been conducted in open session, where the public may observe the proceedings and deliberations. There are committee rules that can be used to close mark-up sessions to all except committee and agency staff, but this is becoming rare, particularly with authorizing committees.

Floor Action

When the full committee has approved a bill, it is ready for a vote by the Senate or House. However, there are several procedural items that precede the actual vote.

In the House, the completed committee bill is sent to the House Committee on Rules. This Committee has the power to establish the length of time for debate and to determine whether floor amendments will be allowed.

Except for House Committee on Rules review, procedures are generally similar in the House and Senate. The bill is placed on a calendar and given a calendar number. In the Senate there are two major calendars, whereas there are five in the House. The House Union Calendar is used to list bills that provide for revenue raising, general appropriations, and general authorizations. The House Calendar is used most often for public bills and resolutions that do not raise revenue or appropriate or authorize funds.

The House Private Calendar is for bills of a private nature, such as claims against the government. There are also a Consent Calendar for noncontroversial bills and a Discharge Calendar that is used only rarely to force action on a measure that has been held up in committee against the wishes of a majority of the House. Bills placed on a calendar are voted on in order of numerical sequence, although both Houses have established procedures to bypass this sequence for speedy consideration of a particular measure.

A bill may be further amended during the floor debate, but because of the need to rely on committee conclusions and expertise, amendments on the floor need considerable support for favorable passage.

When a bill has been passed, it is sent to the other chamber for action, where the entire legislative process starts over.

Often, both the Senate and the House will consider bills of a similar nature. It is unlikely that both will pass identical bills. If they do, the bill is then sent to the White House for action. Usually, the bills will differ, and a conference will be arranged to resolve the differences.

Conference Committee

When differences occur, the house that is holding the bill may request a conference with the other house to settle the issues. Conferees or managers, appointed by the Presiding Officer of the Senate and the Speaker of the House, are generally the ranking members of the committees that have reported the bills, but designated sponsors of major amendments to the bills also may be appointed to the conference committee.

During conference, each house has one vote irrespective of the number of conferees appointed. Conferees are limited during their deliberations to consideration of the matters in disagreement between the two versions of the bill. Furthermore, conferees generally cannot exceed the bounds set in the passed bills. For example, if one house authorized expenditures of $30 million and the other $20 million, a final amount would generally be between $20 and $30 million; $19 million or $31 million would not be acceptable.

When agreement has been reached, a conference report is written that embodies the bill with the conferees' recommendations. Each house then votes on the report. If no agreement is reached by the conferees or should either house not accept the conference report, the bill dies in conference.

Presidential Action

When a bill is sent to the White House, the President has four options. First, he may sign the bill. It immediately becomes law and is sent to the Government Printing Office for publication. Second, he may veto the bill within 10 days (not including Sundays and federal holidays) and return it to Congress. If this action is taken, the Constitution requires him to submit a statement describing his objections. Third, he may allow the bill to become law without his signature. This occurs if he takes no action for 10 days when Congress is in session. His last option is the pocket veto. This occurs if Congress passes a bill near the end of its Second Session and then adjourns before the President has had 10 days to return the bill should he wish to veto it. In this instance, the bill automatically will not become law. Hence, if the President objects to a measure passed at or near the close of a Congress, he may pocket the bill until after adjournment, thus allowing it to die.

If the President vetoes a bill, he must return it to the originating house. At this point, two thirds of the members present and voting affirmatively, which constitutes a quorum, may override the veto. The bill is then sent to the other house, where the identical procedure must occur. When both houses override the veto, the bill becomes law. Should this not occur, the President's veto remains in force.

If a bill becomes law, it is then ready to be considered for funding.

Appropriations Process

The appropriations process is very similar to the authorization process. A few distinct events usually must occur before review by the Committee on Appropriations.

First, a program must be authorized. Therefore, the authorization process must be complete before appropriations consideration. Second, the President's submission of his budget request initiates the review of programs and the President's proposal by the appropriations committees.

By custom and tradition, appropriations measures originate in the House of Representatives. Upon receipt of the President's budget message, the House Committee on Appropriations and the appropriate subcommittee (in the case of most health programs, the Subcommittees on Labor, Health and Human Services, Education and Related Agencies Appropriations in both House and Senate) begin the process.

The first step is the departmental testimony. Each major program director of the federal government appears before the Committee on Appropriations to defend and justify the President's budget request. Since they are employees of the federal government, the President is their ultimate boss. They must defend his budget regardless of what they think. After this, public witness testimony is held. Any citizen or institution or group may request an opportunity to testify before the Committee on Appropriations. Although this is important, it is much more helpful for constituents and those concerned over funding levels and program direction to meet individually with their own legislators, their staff, and committee members.

After completion of the hearings, the members and staff begin the process of preparing their funding recommendations. The subcommittee level is probably the single most important step in the process. Individuals concerned with achieving a goal should recognize that the subcommittee mark-up levels of funding are generally the levels that the full committee adopts.

Bill or Report?

In addition to funding levels being of ultimate importance, each appropriations bill, which is very technically written, is accompanied by a report that describes in lay terms the programs being funded and, most important, how the funds should be used. Often, the report language is as important as the funding because it expresses the intent of the Committee and provides direction for agency and program directors as to how the appropriated funds are to be spent.

Once the subcommittee has acted, the bill and report are sent to the full committee for adoption or approval. Once approved, the measure is sent to the floor for debate and possible amendments and, finally, approval. After both the Senate and the House approve versions of the bill, a conference committee is appointed. This, in the case of health programs, usually consists of the members from both the Senate and House Subcommittees on Labor, Health and Human Services, Education and Related Agencies Appropriations.

It is in conference that the differences of the two bills are compromised. Once this occurs, the final single bill is sent back to the House for approval and then sent to the Senate. After approval by both bodies, the measure is sent to the President, who then has the same four options available as in the authorization process.

What Is a Typical Appropriations Calendar?

January	President's State of the Union Address and submission of budget to Congress
February	House and Senate begin departmental or federal agency testimony
March	Departmental and federal agency testimony continues
April	Public witness testimony in both House and Senate
May	Preparation for mark-up
June	House subcommittee mark-up
July	House full committee and House floor vote, Senate subcommittee mark-up
August	Senate full committee and Senate floor vote
September	House–Senate conference committee and adoption of conference agreement, presidential signature or veto
October	Beginning of new fiscal year

Source

Congress and Health, 6th ed. Government Relations Handbook Series. New York, National Health Council, 1985

Lobbying for Medical Research

*It is my tax money; I have the right to
help determine how it is spent.*

—Mary Lasker

What Is Lobbying?

America is a nation of advocates. Individually and collectively, we seek to influence
our government to set its priorities in accordance with our own concerns.

People speak out at town meetings or city council sessions for improved highways,
and they talk to school officials about changes they believe are necessary in the
curriculum. They call town hall to say they want more frequent garbage collection or
to ask for more tennis courts or soccer fields.

Many groups of people with common interests join organizations, including groups
as varied as the Pharmaceutical Manufacturers Association, Tobacco Institute, United
Automobile Workers, National Rifle Association, National Organization for Women,
and National Wildlife Federation.

Health issues are not exempt from citizen influence. Voices have been raised to
protect nonsmokers from breathing second-hand smoke. The disabled have spoken out
for designated parking spaces, wheelchair ramps, and elevators in public buildings so
that they can live more independent lives. People who have voiced opinions, requested
assistance, or demanded action may think of themselves as outspoken citizens, but
they are, in fact, lobbyists. The organizations they join to represent their interests may
carry out many functions, including public service, sponsorship of research, financial
aid to the needy, or public and member education, but if the organization advocates
government action of any kind, it is also a lobbying group.

Why Lobby for Medical Research?

When asked, the vast majority of Americans support government funding for medical
research. Few people would favor stinting on spending for programs that may result

in a cure for cancer, a vaccine to prevent AIDS, or a treatment that will end disability from arthritis.

However, we have not had a President in over 20 years who has made medical research a high priority; in fact, recent administrations have often proposed cuts in funding. The nation's major political parties totally ignore medical research in their national platforms, and there are no national candidates who work for and strongly support such programs.

Fortunately, many members of Congress have gained sufficient understanding of the importance of aggressive medical research to maintain viable, if not fully funded, research programs. Most senators and representatives will listen to knowledgeable and enthusiastic constituents who can help them to understand the advances that could be made within the next 5 years—with adequate funding. However, more concerned people must begin to voice their feelings on the need to make medical research one of this nation's highest priorities.

We are in danger of losing our competitive edge in biomedical research. We must begin to think of medical research as a significant part of our national defense. We need an organized medical research lobby to educate decision makers on the importance of medical research.

Who Can Lobby?

Any individual or group with an opinion and the means to express it can lobby. Individual citizens can have an impact on public policy, but groups of like-minded people, and coalitions of groups, can be an even stronger force. Many lobbyists are volunteers; others are the paid staff members of organizations. Professional lobbyists often are hired to advocate the interests of individuals, organizations, coalitions, or businesses.

To be effective, a lobbyist must know how government works and be aware of who is involved in the decision-making process. Knowledge of the best timing for a lobbying effort can add greatly to a lobbyist's success.

Can Tax-Exempt Groups Lobby?

Since 1976, nonprofit organizations have been allowed to spend a portion of their budget on lobbying, without fear of losing their tax-exempt (501)(C)(3) status.

How Does a Lobbyist Get Started?

Anyone who can make a phone call or write a letter already knows how to lobby. The rest is learning how to maximize the effectiveness of the approach.

It helps to know something about the legislator or legislators you are planning to contact. What are their interests? What are their backgrounds? What is their record of support on the issue you are advocating? On which committees do they serve, and what positions do they hold? Who chairs the committee that will be considering the proposal for or against which you are lobbying? Who is leading the opposition?

Much of this information can be provided by the staff and volunteer leadership of an organization if you are lobbying as part of a group effort, but it also helps if you follow your elected representative's voting record in the newspaper. Public libraries have indexes that can help you to locate back issues of newspapers if you need help catching up on the status of a research-related bill you are hoping to see passed. *Congressional Quarterly*, a publication issued weekly, is found in large binders in the reference sections of many public libraries and provides excellent information on voting records of senators and representatives. The "Status of Appropriations" and "Status of Legislation" features of this publication are helpful in keeping track of bills as they travel through the legislative process.

If you want to know your own legislator's position on specific legislation, pick up the telephone and ask a member of his or her staff. Most members have offices in their districts and can be contacted easily. Let your representative's staff know if you want a copy of a pending bill. It can be obtained without cost for constituents, as can copies of reports and hearings.

Talking to people in the community is a good way to learn about your representative's interests and concerns and may help you to approach the topic from a point of

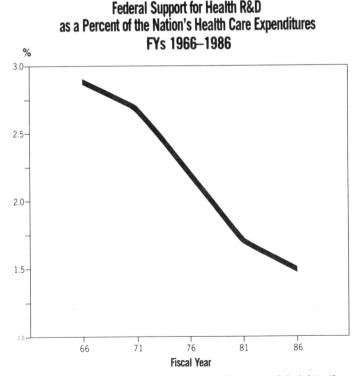

**Federal Support for Health R&D
as a Percent of the Nation's Health Care Expenditures
FYs 1966–1986**

Source: NIH 1986 Data Book. Health Care Financing Administration

mutual interest. A member of Congress who understands the difficulty of caring for a family member with Alzheimer's disease, for instance, may share your concern for research in that area; a senator who has diabetes is likely to understand the importance of research on insulin.

An effective lobbyist knows how the system works. An advocate of increased funding for medical research will want to understand how an appropriations bill moves through the legislature, from introduction to enactment, and will follow its progress from introduction, through committee hearings, and onto the floor of the House and Senate. There are specialized newsletters that track the progress of legislation that affects all aspects of medicine; they are available at many medical libraries, including those operated by county medical societies and medical schools.

Letters, phone calls, and personal visits during this legislative process can help build and maintain interest in the bill. To maximize your effectiveness, be sure contacts are made first with your own congressional representatives and then with members of the committee who will be deliberating your bill. Once the bill is reported out of committee, all members of Congress will play a role in its passage or defeat.

How Can a Lobbyist Get the Facts?

To be effective, a lobbyist needs to know the subject and what impact it will have on members and their constituents. With accurate information, a lobbyist can become known as a helpful and concerned citizen. Without it, such a person lacks credibility.

What will the legislation you are advocating accomplish? Why is it important that it be passed now, instead of next year? What will happen if it does not pass? How much money will it save? How much will not passing it cost—in dollars spent, in lost productivity, or in human lives? What will it do in terms of jobs, numbers of grants, or contracts? What does it mean to various states or districts?

In addition, a representative will want to know how a piece of legislation affects his constituents. How many people in his or her district will be helped by this piece of legislation? Residents of a district with a large number of senior citizens may like to hear that their congressional representative voted for research on arthritis, hearing loss, or Alzheimer's disease. A representative whose constituency consists of many young families may be most interested to learn how research will find new clues to the causes of sudden infant death syndrome or cerebral palsy.

Often the place to get these facts is the headquarters of an organization that advocates your cause; staff or active volunteers may have gathered the facts and figures you need. Other sources of information include public libraries and specialized (including medical) libraries or the government agency that provides the funds for the programs you are advocating.

If you are an expert in a particular area, your input may be of particular value to your legislator. If, for instance, you are a researcher in what you consider to be an underfunded area of medical science or have personal knowledge of what it means to live with a specific disease or disability, let the person whose vote you are trying to influence know this.

How Do Lobbyists Express Their Conviction?

Facts are vital for a lobbyist, but they are not enough. Conviction also is essential. An effective lobbyist sticks to one issue at a time, not advocating medical research one day and preschool education the next. Once your congressional representative's staff members begin to recognize your name and say, "Oh yes, you're with the medical research group," you know they are paying attention to what you have to say.

What Is the Best Way to Write to a Member of Congress?

Today, mail to a member of Congress may be more important than ever. Senators and representatives vote on far more issues than did their predecessors and attend increasingly longer sessions of Congress. Many spend only about 60 days each year in their home districts. Mail is a vital link to the constituents they represent.

Many members and their staffs read all the letters from residents of their district that relate to legislative matters. A staff member may process them initially, but they will almost always be answered, and most members of Congress actually try to read and personally be involved in the replies.

A single thoughtful letter can sometimes change a member's mind or at least convince him or her to review an opinion. Informative letters on an issue can give a good understanding of the thinking of constituents and insight into specific problems.

What Should the Letter Contain?

1. Address your letter properly, and be sure your name, address, and phone number appear on the letter so that the member can respond. Be absolutely certain that names are spelled correctly.

2. Identify the issue or bill. Be as specific as possible and try to give a bill number or a title. Good resources for this information are daily newspapers, specialized newsletters found in medical libraries, or *Congressional Quarterly* in the public library.

3. Write your own congressional representatives or senators or those whose committee assignments or personal interests give them a reason to be interested in the bill. Letters written to all 435 members of the House and 100 senators are often a wasted effort.

4. Be clear. Leave no doubt in the reader's mind where you stand on the issue.

5. Be brief. Letters should be a single page; if more must be said, enclose an attachment elaborating on your single page summary.

6. Be personal. Form letters do not have the same impact as those written by someone who cares enough to take pen in hand or sit down at the typewriter. Give your own reasons for taking a stand.

7. Use facts and figures. See the section on "Major Diseases and Disabilities" later in this book.

8. Be respectful, even if you disagree with your representative's position. Explain why you hope he or she will reconsider.

How Does One Lobby Face to Face?

The first time you meet with a representative or a senator face to face can be exciting, even if you are nervous. Good advance preparation may help to calm your nerves and will make the visit more effective.

1. Call for an appointment. Explain that you are a constituent who has a strong interest in the upcoming medical research funding bill and that you would like to meet with your Congress member to explain your position. If you have specific credentials or experience, explain briefly that this is why you think he or she will want to meet with you. For instance, you may have benefited from an experimental form of cancer therapy, and you want to be sure the program is funded so that others can receive this lifesaving treatment.

2. If appropriate, tell him or her that you are a member of the same political party and that you supported him in the past and/or contributed to his campaign.

3. Be prompt and be brief. Plan to cover your topic in 5 minutes if possible, 10 minutes at most. Do not linger unless your representative or the staff member makes it clear that a longer visit is welcome.

4. Emphasize facts. If you cannot answer a question, admit it and plan to follow up as soon as possible by letter or phone with the information. Within 24 hours, send your host a single-page summary of your position and the most important facts, including the number of people who die from the disease and the number of people afflicted. Such information might be useful in the introduction to a bill or in speeches supporting the bill. Be sure your address and phone number are on the summary sheet so that you can be contacted for further information.

5. Aides *are* influential. Even a firm appointment with a legislator may result in a conversation with an aide instead, due to the great demand on legislators' time. Although it may be more exciting to meet an elected official in person, an interested aide can be an asset to your cause. Present your case to him or her just as if the aide were the representative or senator.

6. Bringing a second interested lobbyist along may make you more comfortable, but more than three people is too many. Do not bring someone along who is not prepared to support the same legislation you are advocating, even if just one of you does most of the talking.

7. Say thank you. Thank your legislator for his or her time when you leave the office. If you feel he or she is sympathetic, offer a financial contribution for his or her campaign. Follow up with a note when you get home. Also write to say thank you if he or she votes the way you asked; most congressional mail asks for favors or expresses complaints, so a thank you letter makes an impression. Be sure to thank the staff person as well.

How Is a Grassroots Network Organized?

Many national organizations have established extensive networks of members who are willing and able to participate in lobbying activities. If such a program has strong leadership and good communication, it can develop a cadre of sophisticated and knowledgeable people who can mobilize influential contacts in a minimal amount of time.

Often called "grassroots" programs, such networks take time, patience, and diligence to develop, but they can coordinate the efforts of many individuals who are lobbying for the same cause and multiply the effectiveness of their efforts.

Key Contacts

The first step in developing a grassroots network is the appointment of key contacts, members who will play major roles in making contacts with participating members, who will aid in the lobbying effort, and who will be looked to as speakers for the organization in a given locality.

Key contacts' responsibilities include developing relationships with elected officials within their areas, keeping lists of members who are willing to send letters, make telephone calls, or make visits to representatives, often on short notice, and maintaining lists of all members in the area with their addresses and phone numbers.

The key contact should be the source of all information to local chapters and serve as a conduit for information to and from the national office. He or she should know the legislative process the group is trying to influence and be prepared to coach interested but inexperienced members in writing letters and talking with representatives.

Key contacts may find it effective to get to know appropriate legislative aides, both locally and nationally. These contacts should also develop local activities in which elected officials can be encouraged to participate, so that the officials will get to know your members and the issues with which you are concerned.

The job of key contact is a demanding one but has great rewards for the person who is committed to obtaining legislative support for an important issue and enjoys playing an active role in the democratic process.

Making It Work

A group of enthusiastic key contacts, scattered throughout the nation, can be a vital force in bringing a message, such as the importance of support for medical research, to the attention of a significant number of legislators. By coordinating their efforts and sharing information, they can eliminate duplication of effort and reach the largest possible number of supporters in Congress.

What Is the Role of a Professional Lobbyist?

Most people contract for consultant services when they do not have the time or the skills to do the job properly themselves. Like lawyers and accountants, professional lobbyists are available for a fee to help you or your organization. Lobbyists are skilled at keeping track of a bill's progress and can tell you when a meeting with your senator or representative would be most effective and the best time to organize a letter-writing campaign.

A lobbyist cannot work magic. He or she cannot invent good reasons for a bill's passage if you do not supply facts or generate enthusiasm. But a lobbyist will be able to help you make the most effective case to the right people at the best time.

One major advantage of hiring a lobbyist is access to important information before it becomes general knowledge. The services of someone who spends full time keeping up on what is happening in government agencies and congressional committees can help volunteers to maximize their effectiveness and help eliminate lost opportunities to have an impact on the system.

Does Lobbying Make a Difference?

The National Institutes of Health began as a one-room laboratory one hundred years ago. The concern of American citizens about the toll taken by illness led to its expansion.

Today, NIH is the world's largest sponsor of biomedical research. This tax-supported agency has done more to eliminate disease and disability than any other institution in the world. Its accomplishments are a tribute to the effectiveness of an organized lobbying effort and citizen participation in the American democratic process.

Promoting Health and Preventing Disease

While it's important to develop new technology to cure disease, one can certainly get a lot more bang for the buck by educating people about how to prevent disease.

— Edwin C. Whitehead
Chairman, Whitehead Associates
Acting Chairman, National Center
for Health Education

What Are Some Goals for Promoting Health and Preventing Disease?

It has become increasingly clear that the solutions to some of the nation's major health problems lie not in the costly medical treatment of disease and disability but rather in a long-term effort to promote health and prevent disease. During the last decade, a shift has begun in our nation's health priorities away from the historically predominant focus on disease treatment toward an emphasis on the policies and resources for promoting health and preventing disease.

The need for alternative approaches was given official recognition in 1979 with publication of *Healthy People*, the United States Surgeon General's first report on health promotion and disease prevention. This report represented the culmination of over a decade of scientific research efforts designed to understand the role of risk factors associated with personal lifestyle and environmental conditions in the causation of disease. Through such research, we have learned that what people eat, how much they exercise, how much they smoke or drink, and what they may be exposed to at work or in the their communities can all affect whether they are likely to achieve their predicted life expectancy and maintain a high quality of life.

The Surgeon General's report established a bold national agenda of five goals for

This article was prepared by John P. Allegrante, Ph.D., Teachers College and School of Public Health, Columbia University, New York, NY.

the significant reduction of disease and premature death and disability in all age groups by 1990:

- A 35 percent reduction in infant mortality to below a level of 9 deaths per 1,000 live births

- A 20 percent reduction in the death rate for children ages 1 to 14 years to below a level of 34 deaths per 100,000 children

- A 20 percent reduction in the death rates for adolescents and young adults ages 15 to 24 years to below a level of 93 deaths per 100,000

- A 25 percent reduction in deaths for adults ages 25 to 64 years to below a level of 400 deaths per 100,000 adults

- A 20 percent reduction in the average annual days of confinement due to acute and chronic conditions in people age 65 and older to an average of 30 or less days per year

To achieve these goals, a national program of health promotion and disease prevention activities was begun in 1980. This program, currently in progress, depends on three major strategies to enable the nation to achieve specific objectives for the reduction of risk factors and the improvement of health by the end of the decade. The strategies include preventive health services, health protection, and health promotion.

What Are Some Preventive Health Services?

Each year, the health of millions of Americans who feel well is threatened because they are unaware of the importance of basic preventive health services or do not know how to gain access to them. Specific age or risk groups should use such services regularly if they are to promote and maintain health and prevent disease. Unwanted pregnancies, unfavorable birth outcomes, childhood infectious diseases, sexually transmitted diseases, and high blood pressure are among the nation's priority health problems. What is being done to reduce substantially the disease, death, and disability associated with these problems?

Family Planning

Because unplanned and unwanted pregnancies can result in problems of growth and development for the infants and disruption of the social and economic status of their mothers, the availability of safe and effective contraception is a critical priority in the delivery of preventive health services.

Pregnancy and Infant Care

To decrease the likelihood of infant low birth weight and mortality at birth, especially among low socioeconomic groups, preventive health services for every pregnant woman should include comprehensive prenatal care, education about the birth process, and continuing postnatal care.

Immunization

Low immunization levels are believed to be responsible for recent epidemics of several of the seven major preventable childhood infectious diseases, such as measles and pertussis, pointing to the need for continuing emphasis on achieving universal childhood immunization.

Control of Sexually Transmitted Diseases

More than 10 million cases of sexually transmitted diseases are diagnosed each year. For this reason, public education policy is focusing on symptoms and treatment, encouraging the use of condoms, screening and early detection in high-risk groups, and providing appropriate treatment of those infected.

High Blood Pressure Control

Elevated blood pressure places millions of Americans, especially black Americans, at risk for coronary heart disease and stroke. The delivery of preventive health services in the community, in the workplace, and in patient care settings now virtually always includes screening and early detection for successful treatment and control of high blood pressure.

What Is Health Protection?

The second major strategy in the nation's broad health promotion and disease prevention effort involves helping communities to provide better health protection for the public. The focus of this effort is on reducing the threats to health by an environment that grows increasingly complex with the rapid social and technologic development of American society. Existing federal laws enacted during the past 20 years, which are enforced by numerous regulatory and other governmental agencies, form the basis for our efforts in health protection. Some of the most important of these are the Environmental Protection Act, the Clean Air Act, the Occupational Safety and Health Act, and the Superfund Act. Current efforts focus on maintaining a healthy physical environment by protecting the public from exposure to toxic agents, occupational health hazards, accidental injury, unsafe air and water, and infectious diseases. There are five national priority areas for prevention through health protection activities that are being conducted at the federal, state, and local levels.

Toxic Agent Control

Efforts are being made to reduce the public's exposure to toxic chemicals and other agents that often are the by-products of America's agricultural, industrial, and technologic development. Such agents include asbestos, petroleum-based contaminants (pesticides), polychlorinated biphenyls (PCBs), toxic gases (radon), and ionizing radiation from nuclear fission energy.

Occupational Safety and Health

Protection of America's workers from exposure to health hazards — carcinogens, asbestos, toxic chemicals, and job-related stress — associated with some types of work is a priority. Workers are being encouraged to promote their health through worksite physical fitness and other lifestyle change programs.

Accident Prevention and Injury Control

Motor vehicle accidents, wounds from firearms, falls, burns, poisonings, and other accidents result in an enormous toll of unnecessary and often preventable injuries and deaths each year. Prevention and control of environmental and other factors is an important component of community health protection efforts.

Fluoridation of Community Water Supplies

Fluoridation of drinking water continues to be the most effective means by which dental caries (tooth decay) can be prevented and is one of the most cost-effective measures we have to protect the health of the general public.

Control of Infectious Diseases

Although infectious diseases are no longer among the leading causes of death, infection by viral, bacterial, and other microbial agents results in millions of disabling and costly illnesses each year. Monitoring, surveillance, and control of such diseases are important activities in our nation's broad prevention strategy.

What Is Being Done to Promote Health?

Whereas disease prevention activities attempt to protect as many people as possible from a potentially health-threatening disease or environmental condition, health promotion — the third major strategy in our national program — seeks to encourage healthy individuals to learn about and adopt lifestyles that are conducive to promoting and maintaining good health. Health promotion is concerned with fostering healthy habits so that people will stop — or never start — smoking or misusing alcohol and drugs, improve their nutrition and physical fitness, and learn to control stress and violent behavior. Activities designed to help people do these things are now offered through the nation's schools, workplaces, hospitals and clinics, and other community settings.

Smoking

Although cigarette smoking — which is believed to be the single most important cause of preventable disease and disability — is declining, helping people to stop smoking and preventing young people from acquiring this health-compromising habit continue to be a major focus of health promotion programming. Legislation to restrict smoking in public places is another aspect of this effort.

Alcohol and Drugs

Alcohol and drug abuse continues to be a major factor in disease, premature death, and disability. Current health promotion efforts combine education, law enforcement, and approaches designed to alter the social acceptability of alcohol and drug use to reduce this problem in the community.

Nutrition

Health promotion to improve the nutritional status of the American population focuses on reducing obesity and the nutritional risk factors (e.g., dietary cholesterol and saturated fat) associated with cardiovascular disease and cancer and on nutrition education to help people select diets that include a wide variety of foods.

Physical Fitness and Exercise

The health effects of regular exercise throughout life have become increasingly evident, and because of the potential benefits of exercise in strengthening the cardiovascular system and helping to reduce or control stress, a priority for health promotion is to continue encouraging Americans to engage in physical fitness activities.

Stress and Violent Behavior

Although stress is an inevitable part of most of our lives, too much stress can have damaging effects on health and can often lead to both physical and emotional illness, violence, and other forms of social pathology. A major aim of health promotion is to reduce stress in our communities and, where possible, to help people learn personal strategies and skills that enable them to better cope with daily stress.

Health Education: The Common Thread

The common theme of the strategies used in our efforts to build a healthy America is education. The goal of health education is to promote and maintain individual and community health through learning and understanding. Through the process of education, we can help people learn about the availability of preventive health services and their appropriate use, raise awareness of environmental threats to community health and the need for adequate health protective legislation, and facilitate the acquisition of knowledge and skills so that individuals can promote their own health through personal lifestyle changes. Ultimately, making available reliable information through education enables people to set priorities and create, along with professionals, solutions for achieving an interest in and a commitment to working toward a common goal of health for all Americans.

Are We Making Progress?

Building a healthier America depends not only on the treatment of disease but also on reducing the consequences of preventable disease and the premature death and disability that Americans suffer each year. Through a well-conceived national program of appropriately targeted preventive health services, health protection activities to reduce exposure to environmental hazards, and health promotion designed to foster greater individual responsibility for health, we are making steady progress toward meeting several of the nation's health objectives. Although the investment of national resources to support research and community demonstration programs in such health promotion and disease prevention efforts has been increasing, we as a nation must be willing to commit additional resources in order to realize the ambitious goal of improving the national health.

Where Can One Obtain More Information on Health Promotion and Disease Prevention?

National Center for Health Education
30 East 29th Street
New York, NY 10016
(212) 689-1886

Office of Disease Prevention and Health Promotion
Public Health Service
U.S. Department of Health and Human Services
Room 2132
330 C Street, S.W.
Washington, DC 20201
(202) 245-7611

Center for Health Promotion and Education
Centers for Disease Control
Building 3, Room 117
Mail Stop A-37
1600 Clifton Road
Atlanta, GA 30333
(404) 329-2838

Source

U.S. Department of Health, Education and Welfare. *Healthy People: The Surgeon General's Report on Health Promotion and Disease Prevention.* DHEW PHS Publication No. 79-55071 Washington, DC, U.S. Government Printing Office, 1979

The Role of Voluntary Health Organizations

Voluntarism is the system of acting freely and in an organized way for the public good and flourishes today with voluntary health agencies meeting the health care needs of Americans.

— Profiles in Health Caring,
National Health Council, 1980

What Are Voluntary Health Agencies?

National voluntary health agencies are organized to combat specific diseases, disabilities, or conditions. They are led by both laypeople and health professionals and are organized on a national basis.

Some have chapters in various states and cities, whereas others have just one national office.

How Did Voluntary Health Agencies Evolve?

Voluntary health agencies evolved from a desire of Americans to help those in need and to contribute to society. Also known as health voluntaries, these agencies provided avenues for people to initiate good will in an era of growing materialism and impersonality in the early 20th century.

Health voluntaries provided the opportunity for individuals to participate in philanthropic institutions and made it possible for those who recognized a health problem to join with others to develop solutions or provide opportunities for services, education, and research.

What Was the First Voluntary Health Agency?

The first voluntary health agency, the National Tuberculosis Association (now the American Lung Association), was founded in 1904. Because it was so successful, similar organizations evolved.

How Many Voluntary Health Agencies Are There in the United States?

There are now hundreds of voluntary health agencies in the United States, but 25 national organizations currently account for the vast majority of programs, volunteers, staff, and expenditures in the voluntary health sector. In addition, there are 80 smaller or emerging agencies. These 105 national agencies have more than 10,000 regional, state, and local units in cities across America.

There are more than 36,000 paid staff nationwide, serving nearly 40 million Americans, and an estimated 18 million volunteers associated with these health voluntaries.

What Are the Major Issues and Concerns of Voluntary Health Agencies?

The primary focus of voluntary health agencies is to reduce and eliminate the incidence and prevalence of specific diseases and conditions.

Agencies that provide patient services work to secure resources to keep pace with increasing health care costs and new medical technologies. This phenomenon has occurred in an era during which government support for service agencies is declining while patient loads are increasing.

Other agencies devote considerable resources to support basic and clinical research. The nation's ongoing explosion of scientific knowledge has created exciting opportunities for research, but funds are not always available to match the opportunities. Many worthwhile efforts remain unfunded.

What Are Voluntary Health Agencies Best Known For?

Voluntary health agencies are best known for their extensive educational efforts in preventing disease and disability and in promoting healthy lives. The antismoking education activities of the American Cancer Society, American Lung Association, and the American Heart Association are well-known examples. They continually seek new ways to motivate people to take better care of themselves, to detect early warning signs, and to seek professional assistance when it is required.

Many voluntary health agencies also disseminate information about current diagnostic, treatment, and rehabilitative advances to health professionals.

Who Benefits Most from Voluntary Health Agencies?

Communities where local affiliates provide direct services to individuals and families in need are the primary beneficiaries of the voluntary health agencies. The extent and type of local service programs are affected by the national agency policy. Other national agency policies affect the proportion of funds that remain in the community

Voluntary Health Agencies

The following are the 1985 levels of support of the 22 member voluntary health agencies of the National Health Council, as published in March 1987 by the National Health Council.

	Public Support	Total support and revenue
	(All numbers are in thousands of dollars)	
American Cancer Society	$242,897	$281,058
American Diabetes Association	20,114	31,290
American Lung Association	77,205	95,013
American Red Cross	283,061	850,727
American Social Health Association	1,227	1,445
Arthritis Foundation	41,387	47,589
Asthma & Allergy Foundation of America	819	912
Cystic Fibrosis Foundation	20,217	20,901
Epilepsy Foundation of America	10,799	16,676
Huntington's Disease Society of America	439	588
Leukemia Society of America	21,793	22,636
Lupus Foundation of America	358	664
March of Dimes Birth Defects Foundation	101,427	107,379
Muscular Dystrophy Association	84,568	90,538
National Council on Alcoholism	699	881
National Easter Seal Society	80,214	197,298
National Foundation for Illeitis and Colitis	3,583	3,674
National Hemophilia Foundation	3,539	6,423
National Multiple Sclerosis Society	35,693	37,124
National Society to Prevent Blindness	6,949	8,260
National Sudden Infant Death Syndrome Foundation	765	785
Tourette Syndrome Association	264	587
Total	$1,038,007	$1,822,448

where the money was raised as well as funds earmarked for distribution by the national organization for use in research and other programs.

Community-based agencies cover a broad range of community health needs. Affiliates participate in solving community health problems, conduct surveys of community resources and needs, stimulate public health departments to be more active, and work with other professional and private organizations in the health field. Local programs range from providing sickroom supplies to operating comprehensive rehabilitation centers.

In What Other Activities Are Voluntary Health Agencies Involved?

Voluntary health agencies have become expert at analyzing health problems and finding solutions. They encourage and support the development of laws and public policies by providing information to document needs and suggest steps for resolving problems. They also influence the administrative structures and procedures of state health, education, and social service departments, advocate budgets for medical and research institutions, and promote local, state, and national governmental health services.

What Is the Relationship Between the Federal Government and Voluntary Health Agencies?

The relationship between the federal government and the health voluntaries varies. Some voluntary health agencies have an explicit policy of not accepting any government funds. Others rely heavily on government reimbursement for services provided, and still others take on special projects with government support or as a modest portion of their ongoing operation. Collaborative programs between the federal government and voluntary health agencies have been developed over the years, such as the High Blood Pressure Program and the Healthy Mother, Healthy Babies Project. Frequently, the government relies on voluntaries to conduct the networking and community outreach necessary to help implement government-sponsored programs.

Do Voluntary Health Agencies Support Research?

Yes, many voluntaries give grants to encourage research in areas related to their mission. Although the greatest number of grants are awarded through the national offices of these agencies, often the state and local affiliates and divisions make such awards as well.

Where Can One Obtain More Information About Voluntary Health Agencies?

National Health Council
622 Third Avenue, 34th Floor
New York, NY 10017-6765
(212) 972-2700

Source

National Health Council

The Role of Animals in Research

Through animal research, we have made remarkable advances in medicine, but we still do not have all the answers. Without continued access to animal models, it is unlikely that cures will be found for such devastating diseases as AIDS, Alzheimer's disease, and heart disease.

— Michael E. DeBakey, M.D.

Why Are Animals Used in Research?

Almost every major medical advance of the last century has depended on research with animals. Animal studies continue to be essential for progress in medicine and health. Without them, we cannot expect significant gains in the prevention and cure of the many illnesses that plague humans and animals. Computer programs, cell cultures, and new laboratory methods have enabled medical researchers to reduce their use of animals for research purposes, but there are few predictions of complete elimination of this practice.

To solve health problems, researchers must use animals, the living systems most closely related to humans. Specific diseases in animals serve as models for understanding the body's defensive response and how the diseases may be treated or prevented. Most people would refuse to submit to an untried surgical procedure or take a medication that had never been tested on a living system. Animals serve as our surrogates in the investigation of human diseases and new ways to treat, cure, or prevent them.

Four major goals of biomedical research with laboratory animals are:

1. To provide fundamental biologic knowledge on which disease prevention and treatment can be based

2. To provide models for the study of actual diseases of humans and animals

3. To test potential therapies, diagnostic and surgical procedures, and medical devices

4. To study the safety and efficacy of new drugs or to determine the potential toxicity of chemicals to which humans and animals will be exposed

How Have We Benefited from Research with Animals?

Later chapters of this book refer to research advances that are saving lives and increasing the ability of disabled people to function. Without the use of animals in medical research, it is unlikely that many of the procedures and treatments we now consider routine medical care would be available to extend life or improve its quality. Some of these accomplishments include:

- Vaccines to prevent polio and rubella

- Rehabilitation for stroke victims

- Insulin treatment for diabetes

- Dialysis for people whose kidneys do not function

- Surgical replacement of joints of people with arthritis

- Removal of cataracts

- Coronary bypass surgery

- Chemotherapy to fight cancer

- Medications to control a wide range of chronic conditions, including hypertension, asthma, epilepsy, schizophrenia, and depression

How Do Animals Benefit from the Research?

Research involving animals has produced major medical breakthroughs in veterinary medicine. Among benefits to animals from research in animals are:

- Vaccines against rabies, distemper, parvovirus, cholera, anthrax, and other diseases in animals

- Treatment of parasitic diseases

- Nutrition research for pet food

- Artificial joints for dogs with hip dysplasia

- Orthopedic surgery for pets and livestock

- Treatment for leukemia in animals

- Genetic research
- Treatment for vitamin deficiency
- Detection and control of tuberculosis in cattle

How Are Laboratory Animals Obtained?

Approximately 90 percent of all research animals are rats, mice, and other rodents bred specifically for this purpose by licensed suppliers. Large animals, such as pigs, cattle, and sheep, are supplied from agricultural sources or private companies. Most nonhuman primates now used in research come from scientific breeding centers, not from the wild. Many cats and dogs used for research are bred for this purpose; others are from public pounds and animal shelters. Of the more than 15 million cats and dogs left in pounds each year, less than 2 percent are used in research.

What Is Being Done To Reduce the Use of Animals in Medical Research?

A National Academy of Sciences report noted a 40 percent drop in the number of animals used for research in the United States between 1968 and 1978. This decrease has been attributed to more efficient use of animals, better methods of animal care, and increased use of nonanimal models. The National Institutes of Health's Division of Research Resources supports research specifically aimed at further reducing the use of animals in research wherever possible.

Nonanimal models are used widely today in the initial screening of chemical substances for potentially harmful effects. Cell and tissue cultures help identify the potential toxicity or medical benefits of chemical compounds in the early stages of investigation, thus greatly reducing the number of animals required for research. However, compounds must also be tested on living systems made up of interrelated organs and organ systems before they can be tried in human beings. Computers and mathematical models can offer insight into those qualities of an organism that can be quantified, but such models cannot, for example, mimic the flow of blood to and from the heart or simulate the function of the brain and nervous system. Current knowledge of the complexities of higher organisms is still quite primitive. Scientists cannot create an organ or even a single cell. Therefore, the replacement of complete animals with nonanimal models for much advanced basic biomedical research is an unlikely prospect for the foreseeable future.

How Are Research Animals Protected?

An extensive system of laws, guidelines, regulations, and principles helps to ensure the welfare of laboratory animals. The Animal Welfare Act is a federal law that sets standards for the care and treatment of laboratory animals, including housing, feeding, cleanliness, ventilation, and veterinary care. It covers all species used in medical research, with the exception of rats and mice. The law assigns responsibility for administration and enforcement to the United States Department of Agriculture and details procedures for registration, recordkeeping, and reporting on the number and uses of research animals.

The National Institutes of Health have stated that the proper use and welfare of research animals is among its highest priorities. Every biomedical research institution that receives grants from the NIH must have an animal care and use committee and is expected to follow the recommendations set forth in the Animal Resources Program Branch's 70-page booklet, *Guide for the Care and Use of Laboratory Animals.* The *Guide* is revised regularly to ensure that scientists and research institutions are kept informed of current developments and advanced concepts in laboratory care.

Voluntary accreditation from the American Association of Accreditation for Laboratory Animal Care (AAALAC) is also highly regarded as a check in the system. AAALAC accreditation identifies institutions that offer first-rate animal care.

Do Americans Support the Use of Animals in Research?

The vast majority of Americans do support the use of animals in research. A National Family Opinion Poll survey conducted for the Foundation for Biomedical Research in 1985 shows that 77 percent of the American public support the use of animals in biomedical research. Other key findings include the following:

- 75 percent of the public support government regulations that require product safety testing on animals before human use.

- 70 percent support basic biomedical research, even when it will not lead directly to a disease cure or treatment.

- 65 percent oppose organizations attempting to stop the use of animals in research and testing.

- Most respondents — 57 percent — were unaware of the laws and government regulations currently in effect regarding care and treatment of laboratory animals.

- More than 80 percent of the sample approve of animal testing for new prescription drugs.

Where Can One Obtain More Information on Animals in Research?

Foundation for Biomedical Research
818 Connecticut Ave., N.W.
Suite 303
Washington, DC 20006
(202) 457-0654

The Center for Alternatives to Animal Testing
The Johns Hopkins School of Hygiene and Public Health
615 N. Wolfe Street
Baltimore, MD 21205
(301) 955-3343

Animal Resources Program Branch
Division of Research Resources
National Institutes of Health
Building 31, Room 5B59
9000 Rockville Pike
Bethesda, MD 20892
(301) 496-5175

Source

Foundation for Biomedical Research

How the Body Works

No single part of the body operates in isolation. Move your little finger, and you have put into operation a whole series of events that affect both the nervous and muscular systems.

Diseases and disabling conditions are seldom limited to one system of the body. In order to understand their full impact, it is helpful to be aware of how various systems in the body work.

The systems chosen for inclusion in this book do not, of course, represent all of the body systems. They are the systems that relate most closely to the majority of diseases and disabilities described herein.

The Cardiovascular System

What Is the Cardiovascular System?

The cardiovascular system transports the nutrients, oxygen, and water that are required for the nourishment of all body tissues and removes the carbon dioxide and other waste products that are produced by all cells. It also carries substances produced in one part of the body that are needed elsewhere, such as specialized cells, antibodies used in fighting infection, and hormones. Blood is the vehicle of transport. The pumping of the heart provides the driving force, and the vascular system is the conduit for the blood.

There are really two vascular systems, the pulmonary vasculature through the lungs and the systemic vasculature through the rest of the body. Each starts with a large artery leading from the heart—the pulmonary artery in the pulmonary vasculature and the aorta in the systemic vasculature. These large arteries divide into progressively smaller ones, the smallest of which are arterioles. These feed into the capillaries, where the exchange of gases, water, nutrients, wastes, and other blood-borne substances takes place. Blood from the capillaries drains into tiny venules that join into progressively larger veins that ultimately return to the heart.

What Is the Structure of the Heart?

The heart is in the chest, slightly to the left of the midline. It is about the size of a fist. The heart is almost all muscle, but it also has valves, an electrical conduction system for stimulating the muscle, and a blood supply. Heart muscle (myocardium) is different from other muscles of the body because it can contract repeatedly 60, 80, or even 100 times a minute—for a lifetime—and because it contracts automatically.

The heart is a single structure with four chambers and four valves. It can be thought of as two pumping systems, the right heart and the left heart. In the right heart, blood returning from the body is pumped to the lungs, where excess carbon dioxide is exchanged for oxygen. In the left heart, oxygenated blood returning from the lungs is pumped into the arterial system leading to the body. Both the right heart and the left heart have two chambers, an atrium and a ventricle. The heartbeat results from the contraction of the ventricles. Valves are positioned between each atrium and each ventricle and at the outlet of each ventricle so that with each heartbeat, blood can move only forward into the arterial system and not backward into the atrium.

For example, the mitral valve, which is between the left atrium and left ventricle, closes when the left ventricle begins to contract. As the pressure in the left ventricle increases, it opens the aortic valve and ejects blood into the aorta. The ventricular contraction creates what is called systolic pressure. As the ventricle relaxes, the pressure in it drops, and as soon as it drops below the arterial pressure, the aortic valve closes. This resting phase of the heart is diastole, and the pressure to which the arterial system falls is diastolic pressure. This pulsating blood pressure is described by two numbers, such as 120/80, corresponding to the systolic and diastolic pressures. It is measured in millimeters of mercury, the height of a column of mercury that could be supported by that pressure.

How Does the Heart Function?

The contraction of heart muscle begins with an electrical signal in the right atrium that is conducted along special pathways into and through the ventricles. The natural pacemaker in the right atrium fires repeatedly, once for each heartbeat. The rhythm of the heart is regular, but its rate responds to the return of blood from the periphery, to signals from the brain through the autonomic nervous system, and to blood-borne substances. There can be great changes in heart rate with exercise, but there is also a normal variation with breathing, which can be quite marked in children—an increase with a deep breath in and a decrease on exhaling.

Normal functioning of the heart, as of all parts of the body, depends on an adequate blood supply from three major coronary arteries—the right, the left anterior descending, and the left circumflex—and their progressively smaller branches. The larger arteries are on the outer surface of the heart, and their smaller branches are distributed throughout the heart muscle.

What Are Some Disorders and Diseases of the Cardiovascular System?

The inner surface and inner layers of an artery may become thickened and otherwise changed in a process called "atherosclerosis." The result is narrowing and hardening (arteriosclerosis), with a decrease in the amount of blood that can flow through the artery. When the coronary arteries are involved, the result is coronary or ischemic heart disease, the most common form of heart disorder. When a coronary artery is seriously narrowed, the amount of blood that can flow to the heart muscle may not meet the needs of an extra workload, as during exercise. Typically, exertion will result in a squeezing pain in the chest that may radiate into the left arm and elsewhere but

The heart beats between 70 and 80 times per minute, or about 100,000 times per day. While you rest or sleep, your heart pumps about 2½ ounces (70 milliliters) of blood with each beat. It may not sound like much, but it adds up to nearly 5 quarts (approximately 5 liters) of blood pumped by the heart in one minute, or about 75 gallons (300 liters) per hour.

The output of the heart can vary according to the body's needs. For example, during periods of vigorous exercise, when the body demands more oxygen- and nutrient-rich blood, the heart can increase its output by nearly five times.

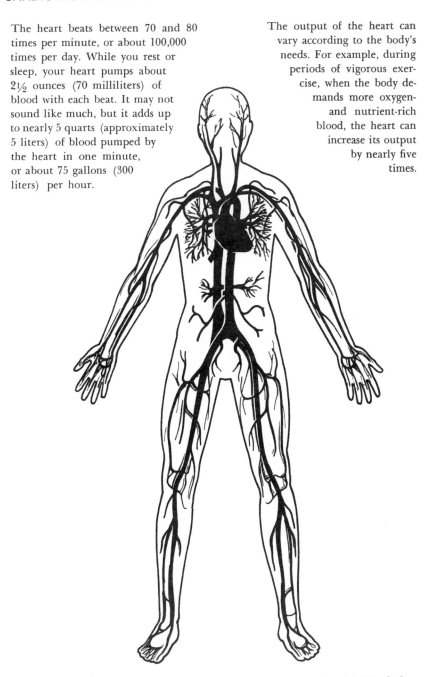

A vast web of blood vessels supplies all areas of the body with blood. Some blood vessels carry fresh, oxygen-rich blood (shown in red); some carry used, oxygen-poor blood (in blue). The pumping heart keeps the blood moving through the vessels—so that blood in the heart can travel to the big toe and back in less than 60 seconds.

Source: National Heart, Lung, and Blood Institute, NIH

then disappears shortly after exercise stops. Such an episode is a temporary inadequacy of blood flow, or ischemia, and the pain it produces is called "angina pectoris."

A narrowed coronary artery may become blocked completely because of a blood clot. When this happens, the downstream heart muscle fails to get enough blood to survive even under its normal workload. In a few hours, it undergoes irreversible damage and then scar formation. This is a heart attack, or myocardial infarction.

When heart muscle fails to get adequate blood or when there is scar tissue, the heart no longer pumps as effectively. This may result in an inadequate supply of blood to the body, where the most serious damage may occur in such organs as the brain and kidneys, or blood may back up in organs from which it should be returning freely to the heart, causing congestion of the lungs and the liver and collection of fluid in the tissues (edema). This may develop gradually and last a long time, as in chronic congestive heart failure, or it can appear suddenly with a heart attack and such catastrophic results as cardiogenic shock and death.

Heart disorders can affect the heart valves so that they fail to open completely (narrowing or stenosis) or fail to close completely (leaking, insufficiency, or regurgitation). Any valve may be affected, but those on the left side—the mitral and aortic valves—are much more commonly involved. Valve disorders may be due to a birth defect (congenital) or, more commonly, may be acquired as a result of rheumatic fever, calcium deposits, the loss of valve supports, or infection.

Heart muscle, like other muscles in the body, enlarges when it has to work consistently against an extra load. When there is high blood pressure, the left ventricle has an extra load continuously, and it enlarges, or undergoes hypertrophy. Hypertrophy may also occasionally develop without a known cause. Heart muscle can also stretch abnormally; the result is cardiomegaly, a dilated and enlarged heart.

Other diseases of the heart include primary disorders of the heart muscle (cardiomyopathies) generally due to unknown causes, inflammation of the heart (myocarditis), infection involving the heart valves or the interior surfaces of the heart (endocarditis), and infection or inflammation involving the external surface and sac surrounding the heart (pericarditis). The heart muscle can be affected by disorders that primarily involve other organs of the body. Congenital abnormalities can involve the valves and the structure of the heart chambers, particularly the walls that separate the right and left chambers, and the great vessels that connect to the heart or to each other.

Veins are thin-walled vessels. Many veins have valves to help maintain the return of blood to the heart against the force of gravity. If these valves give out, the result is varicose veins, the marked dilatation of the larger veins. Another complication, thromboembolism or the development of blood clots, may affect the venous system. This can produce symptoms where it occurs, but even more seriously, clots may break off and be carried to the lungs, where they can obstruct blood flow.

Arteries or, less often, veins may become dilated and form an aneurysm. This blood-filled pocket or sac most often occurs on the aorta, abdominal arteries, and arteries at the base of the brain. The condition is dangerous because of the possibility that the aneurysm may rupture.

Disorders of the regularity of the heartbeat are called "arrhythmias." In the absence of heart disease, they are not a serious problem, but if they are caused by heart disease, they can be life-threatening, causing ventricular fibrillation, ineffective contractions of the ventricles without pumping blood.

How Can the Cardiovascular System Be Protected?

A healthy cardiovascular system is vital for overall well-being. Good health habits, including not smoking, treating high blood pressure, and maintaining normal blood cholesterol, are important ways to maintain this system. Related factors include a balanced diet, normal body weight, and regular exercise.

Where Can One Obtain More Information on the Cardiovascular System?

National Heart, Lung, and Blood Institute
National Institutes of Health
Building 31, Room 4A21
Bethesda, MD 20892
(301) 496-4236

American Heart Association
7320 Greenville Ave.
Dallas, TX 75231
(214) 750-5300

Glossary

Capillaries. Tiny blood vessels that distribute blood carrying oxygen throughout the body
Coronary care unit. An emergency mobile or hospital facility equipped with monitoring devices and staffed with specially trained personnel
Defibrillator. An electronic device that helps reestablish normal contraction rhythms in a malfunctioning heart
Digitalis. A drug used to treat congestive heart failure and sometimes used to treat certain arrhythmias
Myocardium. This muscular heart wall contracts to pump blood out of the heart and then relaxes, allowing the heart to refill with blood

Sinus node. The heart's natural pacemaker, located in the top of the heart's right atrium; this group of specialized cells generates the electrical impulses that cause the heart to contract

Source

National Heart, Lung, and Blood Institute

The Endocrine System

What Is the Endocrine System?

The endocrine system is the body's regulator. Its cells and glands secrete chemical messengers, known as hormones, into either surrounding tissues or the bloodstream.

How Does the Endocrine System Work?

The endocrine system has three parts. The first is the tissues that produce and secrete the hormones. The second is the environment through which the hormones travel. And the third is the target tissues upon which the hormones act. Endocrine disorders occur when too much or too little of a hormone is produced or when there is an abnormal response to a hormone by the target tissue.

Many tissues in the body produce and secrete hormones. This is the sole function of the pituitary, thyroid, parathyroid, and adrenal glands and of the islets of the pancreas. Hormone production and secretion are but one of many functions of the ovaries, testes, hypothalamic region of the brain, heart, gastrointestinal tract, and kidneys.

Over 50 hormones are known to exist, and undoubtedly others are yet to be discovered. Some are produced by only a single type of cell in a single tissue; for example, insulin is produced by the pancreatic islets and growth hormone by the anterior pituitary gland. Others, in contrast, are produced by many tissues. Hormones vary widely in their structure, too. Some, such as the major adrenal, ovarian, and testicular hormones, are slightly modified forms of the simple dietary constituent, cholesterol; others are very large proteins, consisting of hundreds of amino acids.

Hormones act on tissues both very near to and distant from where they are produced. Some hormones enter the bloodstream but travel only a short distance; for instance, the hypothalamic (brain) hormones travel a fraction of an inch to reach their targets in the pituitary gland. Some are carried in the bloodstream to a limited number of targets; for example, parathyroid hormone acts on the kidneys and bone to promote conservation of calcium. Other hormones, such as thyroxine, cortisol, and insulin, are carried by the bloodstream throughout the entire body to act on many tissues.

This article was prepared by Robert D. Utiger, M.D., School of Medicine, University of North Carolina at Chapel Hill, and a member of the Endocrine Society.

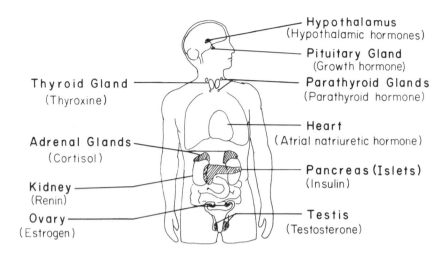

Hormones that act in the tissue where they are produced include estrogen and testosterone. In the ovary, estrogen produced immediately adjacent to the growing ovum (egg) is vitally important for the maturation of the ovum, and testosterone produced in the testis acts within that tissue to stimulate sperm formation. These two hormones also act in other tissues to influence female and male sexual characteristics and behavior.

All cells in the body are exposed to hormones. The ability of cells to respond to a specific hormone depends on whether or not they have receptors for that hormone, and thus the presence or absence of appropriate receptors on the target cells is a critical determinant of hormone action.

What Is the Function of Hormones?

Hormones carry information within a tissue and from one tissue to another. They regulate many different physiologic functions. They are essential for normal reproductive processes in both women and men, for maintenance of pregnancy once conception has occurred, and for milk production for infant nurture. They govern growth and development during childhood and repair of injury throughout life. They play a critical role in maintaining the body's internal environment through their ability to regulate intake and loss of water, salt, and calcium. Hormones also are necessary for normal energy metabolism, since they determine the rates at which such foods as sugar, fat, and protein are used or stored.

What Are Some Endocrine Diseases?

The most common endocrine disorder is diabetes mellitus. Diabetes results in high levels of sugar in the blood but starvation within tissues because sugar is not properly processed so that it can enter them. Diabetes is due either to production of too little insulin or to lack of response of target tissues to the action of insulin. It occurs in both children and adults and may result in an acute life-threatening illness (diabetic ketoacidosis) or cause a wide variety of chronic problems, such as loss of vision, kidney failure, and neurologic and vascular disease.

Other common endocrine disorders are female and male infertility, osteoporosis, increased thyroid hormone production (hyperthyroidism), thyroid hormone deficiency (hypothyroidism), enlargement of the thyroid gland (goiter), and short stature. These disorders can often be diagnosed and treated using modern diagnostic techniques and treatment programs.

Where Can One Obtain More Information on the Endocrine System?

Office of Health Research Reports
National Institute of Diabetes and Digestive and Kidney Diseases
Building 31, Room 9A04
National Institutes of Health
Bethesda, MD 20892
(301) 496-3583

Endocrine Society
9650 Rockville Pike
Bethesda, MD 20814
(301) 571-1802

Glossary

Atrial natriuretic hormone. Lowers blood pressure and promotes salt loss in urine
Cortisol. Regulates tissue metabolism, enhances adaptation to stress
Estrogen. Stimulates sexual development and fertility in women
Growth hormone. Stimulates growth of the skeleton and other tissues
Hypothalamic hormones. Regulate secretion of growth hormone and other hormones
    from the pituitary gland
Insulin. Stimulates use of sugar in many tissues
Parathyroid hormone. Maintains blood calcium and bone integrity
Renin. Increases blood pressure and retention of salt
Testosterone. Stimulates sexual development and fertility in men
Thyroxine. Stimulates oxygen consumption and energy production

The Immune System

What Is the Immune System?

The immune system is a complex network of organs, cells, and specialized substances distributed throughout the body that protect the body from infection or disease. The immune system fights off infections by such agents as bacteria and viruses. When the immune system malfunctions or breaks down, a wide variety of diseases, from allergy to multiple sclerosis to arthritis to cancer, can result.

How Does the Immune System Work?

The immune system defends the body with an elaborate regulatory-communications network of cells, organized into sets and subsets that receive and distribute information. This results in a prompt, appropriate, and effective immune response.

The immune system is able to distinguish between self and nonself and is able to remember previous experiences and react accordingly. Once you have had mumps, your immune system will prevent you from getting it again—you have been immunized.

What Is an Antigen?

An antigen is a substance foreign to the body (any of the millions of nonself molecules) that stimulates the production of antibodies by the immune system. A virus, a bacterium, a fungus, a parasite, or even a portion or product of one of these organisms can be an antigen.

What Are the Major Organs of the Immune System?

The major organs of the immune system throughout the body are called "lymphoid" organs because they are concerned with the growth, development, and deployment of lymphocytes, the white cells that are the key operatives of the immune system. Lymphoid organs include the bone marrow, the thymus, the lymph nodes, and the spleen, as well as the tonsils, the appendix, and elevated areas of tissue (Peyer's patches) in the small intestine.

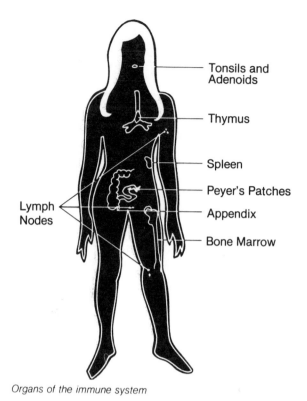

Organs of the immune system

Source: Understanding the Immune System. NIH Publication 84-529, 1983

What Is an Immune Deficiency Disease?

An immune deficiency disease results when the immune system lacks one or more components. These diseases can be inherited, acquired through illness, or produced as an inadvertent side effect of certain drug treatments.

People with advanced cancer may have immune deficiencies as a result of the disease process. Transient immune deficiencies can develop in the wake of common viral infections, including influenza, mononucleosis, and measles. Immune responsiveness can also be depressed by blood transfusions, malnutrition, and stress.

AIDS is such a serious disease because it attacks the infected person's immune system, allowing opportunistic infections to develop, since the body cannot defend itself against them.

Why Is Research on the Immune System So Vital?

The immune system plays a major role in human health and disease. It is only in the last several decades that scientists have begun to uncover its secrets. Immunologists will continue to gain insight into possible ways to manipulate the chemical mechanisms of the immune system so that someday they may be able to adjust its components,

stimulating the malfunctioning ones into effective action and depressing the hyper-
activity of others. Immunology is an exciting and fast-moving discipline and vital to
all biomedical research.

How Have We Benefited from Intense Immune System Research?

The field of immunology has been developing rapidly over the past decade because
of scientific research supported by the National Institute of Allergy and Infectious
Diseases and other organizations. This rapid expansion of knowledge is augmented
enormously by the linking of immunology with numerous other disciplines and by
increasingly sophisticated biotechnology.

Much of the AIDS research conducted by the National Institute of Allergy and
Infectious Diseases and the National Cancer Institute is directed toward restoring or
enhancing the immune system of those infected with the AIDS virus. The knowledge
and experience gained through this effort will benefit all those with immune deficiency
diseases, whatever the cause.

Where Can One Obtain More Information on the Immune System?

National Institute of Allergy and Infectious Diseases
Office of Research Reporting and Public Response
National Institutes of Health
Building 31, Room 7A32
Bethesda, MD 20892
(301) 496-5717

American Academy of Allergy and Immunology
611 East Wells Street
Milwaukee, WI 53202
(414) 272-6071

Joint Council of Allergy and Immunology
P.O. Box 520
Mt. Prospect, IL 60056-3386
(312) 255-1024

Glossary

Allergen. Any substance that causes an allergy
Allergy. The inappropriate and harmful response of the immune system to a normally
    harmless substance

Antibody. Protein molecules produced and secreted by certain types of white cells in response to stimulation by an antigen

Antigen. Any substance that provokes an immune response when introduced into the body

Appendix. An organ of the immune system

Autoantibody. An antibody that reacts against a person's own tissue

Autoimmune disease. A disease that results when the body's immune system produces harmful autoantibodies

B cells. White blood cells of the immune system derived from bone marrow and involved in the production of antibodies, also called B lymphocytes

Bone marrow. Soft tissue located in the cavities of the bones responsible for producing blood cells

Epitope. A characteristic shape or marker on an antigen's surface

Helper T cells. A subset of T cells that start antibody production

Immune complex. Large molecules formed when antigen and antibody bind together

Immune response. The activity of the immune system against foreign substances

Immunocompetent. Able to develop an immune response

Lymph nodes. Small bean-sized organs of the immune system, distributed widely throughout the body

Monoclonal antibodies. Antibodies specific for only one antigen

Parasite. A plant or animal that lives, grows, and feeds on or within another living organism

Severe combined immunodeficiency disease (SCID). A disease in which infants are born lacking all major immune defenses

Spleen. An organ in the abdominal cavity that is an important site of antibody production

Subunit vaccine. A vaccine produced from any part of an infectious agent

Suppressor T cells. Subset of T cells that stop antibody production

T cells. White blood cells that are processed in the thymus

Thymus. A central lymphoid organ important in the development of immune capability

Vaccine. A substance that contains the antigen of an organism

Virus. Submicroscopic microbe causing infectious disease that can reproduce only in living cells

Sources

Understanding the Immune System. Bethesda, MD, NIH Publication No. 84-529, October 1983

National Institute of Allergy and Infectious Diseases

The Nervous System

What Is the Nervous System?

The nervous system is comprised of the brain, the spinal cord, and the nerves that travel to and from all parts of the body. Nerves connect the brain and spinal cord with the sensory organs, muscles and skin, and all the organs in the body.

The central nervous system allows us to think, move our muscles, and control automatic functions, such as breathing and pumping blood. We also use the nervous system to gather new information from the eyes, ears, and other sense organs and to integrate this information with what we have already learned. The peripheral nervous system branches out to the tips of our fingers and toes from the main connections along the central nervous system. Messages to and from the peripheral nervous system must connect with the central nervous system to be understood and voluntarily acted on.

How Does the Nervous System Work?

The nervous system is made up of trillions of cells. The most important of these are the nerve cells, or neurons, the workhorses of the nervous system. The system also contains glial cells that fill spaces between nerve cells, vascular cells that make up the nervous system's blood vessels, and connective tissue cells that line the surface of the brain.

The nerve cell is the basic unit of communication within the body. Neurons in the brain and other parts of the nervous system carry messages to and from each other, muscles and organs, and the environment to help the body perform its many functions. Each neuron has a cell body where the nucleus that maintains the cell's life is found. Many branchlike filaments, called dendrites, sprout from the nerve cell body to receive messages from other nerve cells. One long axon extends away from the cell body toward another nerve cell, muscle, or organ.

Nerve cells communicate with each other through an electrochemical process. An electrical message generated within the nerve cell passes through the cell body and travels the length of the axon to the axonal tip, where it stimulates the release of chemicals known as "neurotransmitters." These neurotransmitters are released into the synapse, the tiny gap that separates one nerve cell from another. Crossing this gap, the neurotransmitters lock onto receptors on a neighboring cell's dendrites. This rendezvous of neurotransmitters and receptors sparks a second electrical message that travels along other nerve cells until it reaches its target and carries out an action: you inhale, for example, or move your finger.

However, not all receiving nerve cells fire after neurotransmitters find receptors. One nerve cell may have thousands of receptors capable of receiving conflicting messages from hundreds of other cells. Some neurotransmitters (excitatory) may tell the receiving nerve to fire while others (inhibitory) may modify the fire command. The particular mix of excitatory and inhibitory neurotransmitters determines if firing takes place and if messages are relayed or stopped.

What Is the Function of the Brain?

The brain orchestrates behavior, movement, feeling, sensing—even breathing and blood pressure. Without it, you cannot fall in love, lift a pencil, or enjoy a concert. The brain is divided into two hemispheres. Some brain functions, such as hearing and vision, are served by both hemispheres, but certain activities originate in one side or the other. The left hemisphere, for example, controls movement and receives sensations from the right side of the body. The right hemisphere controls those same functions on the body's left side. Generally, the left hemisphere controls language.

Each hemisphere is divided into four lobes. The frontal lobe and the temporal lobe help you regulate your behavior and learn new things. Without the frontal lobe, you could not plan a picnic or decide to move indoors when a rainstorm threatens. The temporal lobe is the seat of memory and strong emotions; your first kiss is stored there, but that is also where the pangs of jealousy originate. The parietal lobe receives information from the eyes, ears, nose, and tongue and sends messages to move muscles. This is also the part of the brain that helps you mimic and orients you in space; you use the parietal lobe to repeat words after your French teacher or to navigate from a road map. At the back of the head, the occipital lobe coordinates vision. Near the base of the brain lies the cerebellum, which helps coordinate movement. Were it not for the cerebellum, you would not be able to run, walk, or even step off a curb without falling over. It also lets you perform intricate movements, such as threading a needle and buttoning your shirt.

What Are Some Disorders of the Central Nervous System?

At least 650 disorders have been identified as "neurologic" or "communicative." There are the developmental disorders that begin in childhood: cerebral palsy, spina bifida, autism, Tay-Sachs disease, Batten's disease, Tourette syndrome, learning disorders, lipid storage disorders, and numerous other birth defects and genetic disorders that affect the nervous system. There are many different types of epilepsy. There are atrophic disorders, such as amyotrophic lateral sclerosis (ALS), and all kinds of neuromuscular disorders, including myasthenia gravis, the muscular dystrophies, and multiple sclerosis.

Stroke, a cerebrovascular accident, is the third leading cause of death in the United States. Survivors often suffer loss of language (aphasia) and other lasting disabilities. Spinal cord injury and head injury, too, traumatize the nervous system, often permanently.

Such disorders as Alzheimer's disease, Huntington's disease, and now AIDS dementia are major national health concerns. Demyelinating disorders—perhaps the best known is multiple sclerosis—continue to cause disabilities as scientists seek to understand their origins and mechanisms.

Hearing loss is among the most commmon and serious problems in the United States; it affects both children and adults, as do disorders of speech and language.

How Prevalent Are Nervous System Disorders?

Based on estimates from voluntary agencies and experts in relevant fields, the major neurologic and communicative disorders collectively affect 42.6 million Americans. An estimated 2 million living Americans have suffered a stroke. Epilepsy, too, is present in 2 million people, and 1 million people have experienced head and spinal cord injuries.

There are today over 3 million Americans with Alzheimer's disease and other types of dementia, and that number is increasing as the population ages and as more cases of AIDS dementia are identified. About 2 million people are profoundly deaf; another 15 million have partial deafness. Those with speech and language problems now number 10 million. Movement disorders, such as Parkinson's and Huntington's diseases, affect half a million people, and a million Americans have neuromuscular disorders.

What Kind of Research Is Being Done?

Neuroscience research can be divided into two broad categories: basic research aimed at understanding how the central nervous system works and clinical research involving patients and seeking new knowledge about specific disorders. Basic research gives us the information we need to apply to particular neurologic and communicative problems. Clinical research provides the ultimate payoff in improved methods of therapy and prevention. Each type of research is essential.

There are hundreds of basic investigations in progress today. Scientists involved in basic studies of the nervous system are steadily discovering new neurotransmitters and identifying their full functions to help explain their roles in disease. The neurotransmitters acetylocholine, dopamine, and GABA have been linked to Alzheimer's disease, Parkinson's disease, and Huntington's disease, respectively.

Other substances under study enhance cell growth. Scientists think that these substances, called "trophic factors," may hold the key to regenerating damaged nerve cells, thereby reversing the effects of, for example, spinal cord injury.

Genetic studies are yielding discovery after discovery. Scientists recently identified gene markers for Huntington's disease, Duchenne muscular dystrophy, and neurofi-bromatosis. Tests are now available or being developed to detect these disorders. While scientists in many disciplines seek viable strategies for repairing or replacing defective genes, diagnostic and carrier tests have value for people at risk.

New information about brain function is emerging from studies involving imaging technology, such as positron emission tomography (PET) and magnetic resonance imaging (MRI). These technologies allow scientists to study the brain in living patients without surgery. A major advance achieved through the use of PET was visualization of receptors for dopamine—the neurotransmitter deficient in Parkinson's disease.

Much of the clinical research being done today is designed to determine the safety and effectiveness of new drugs or surgical treatments. Four new anticonvulsant drugs developed through research are now available to epilepsy patients, and others are in various stages of testing. Some stroke-prone patients are being spared the risk and expense of surgery since research demonstrated that aspirin combined with blood pressure control is just as effective in preventing stroke. Studies have also shown that widely used decongestant and antihistamine drugs are not effective treatments for otitis media, a common childhood ear infection, and have demonstrated the value of the antibiotic amoxicillin. Advances in technology have enabled investigators to develop a cochlear implant that allows the profoundly deaf to hear sound and a prosthetic device that restores bladder function in many disabled people.

How Much Is Being Spent on Research on Nervous System Disorders?

Within the federal government, the focal point for biomedical research on the brain and nervous system, including studies of the senses of communication, is the National Institute of Neurological and Communicative Disorders and Stroke (NINCDS), a part of the National Institutes of Health. In fiscal year 1986, the NINCDS spent $414.4 million for basic and clinical research on the brain and central nervous system. Basic research accounted for almost 22 percent of the budget ($89.6 million); about 78 percent ($324.8 million) went for research on specific disorders.

Other federal agencies that support research on the nervous system include the National Institute on Aging, the National Institute of Mental Health, and the Veterans Administration. In addition, there are numerous private sources of funding for neuro-science research; chief among them are the nation's voluntary health organizations and private foundations dedicated to the conquest of nervous system diseases.

What Is the Research Outlook?

Research on the nervous system is under way in laboratories and clinics around the world. Watch for research scientists to develop safer, more effective drugs for neu-rologic diseases, to unlock the mysteries of memory, to find ways to correct or replace

OUR KNOWLEDGE OF THE NEURON

20 Years
Ago

Today

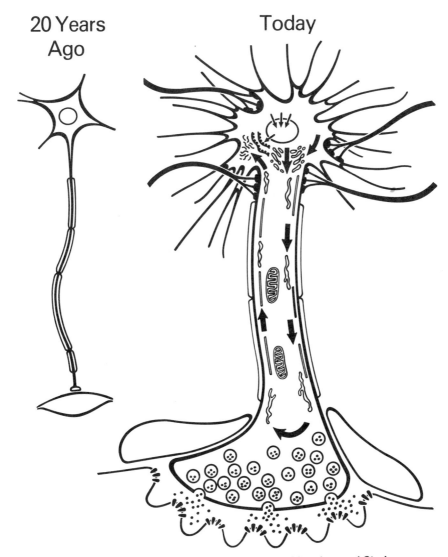

Source: National Institute of Neurological and Communicative Disorders and Stroke

defective genes, to expand studies involving tissue implants into the brain, to develop more sensitive hearing aids, to learn how the AIDS virus damages the nervous system, to regrow neurons in the damaged spinal cord. New ways of viewing the brain, new discoveries about how the nervous system works, and new animal models of human disease have made such exciting research possible that many scientists expect the latter years of the 20th century to be the "Decade of the Brain."

Where Can One Obtain More Information on the Nervous System?

National Institute of Neurological and Communicative Disorders and Stroke
National Institutes of Health
Building 31, Room 8A16
Bethesda, MD 20892
(301) 496-5751

Glossary

Dendrites. The branchlike portions of a nerve cell that conduct impulses to the body
   of the cell
Epilepsy. A group of neurologic disorders characterized by uncontrolled electrical
   discharge from the nerve cells of the cerebral cortex
Dementia. Impairment in mental function and cognitive abilities in an alert individual
Glia. The cells that comprise the supporting tissue of the brain and spinal cord
Neurons. The nervous system's basic cells; carriers of nerve impulses
Neurotransmitter. A chemical messenger used by the nervous system to move nerve
   signals from one nerve cell to another

Source

National Institute of Neurological and Communicative Disorders and Stroke

Major Illnesses
and Disabilities

AIDS

What Is AIDS?

AIDS, or acquired immunodeficiency syndrome, is the final stage of a series of health problems caused by a virus known as HIV (human immunodeficiency virus). The virus attacks the white blood cells (T lymphocytes) that are responsible for fighting infection, damaging the person's immune system. The person then becomes vulnerable to a variety of infections by bacteria, protozoa, fungi, other viruses, and malignancies, which may cause such life-threatening illnesses as pneumonia, meningitis, and cancer. These infections are called "opportunistic diseases" because they are conditions that would not get a foothold in a healthy person but have an opportunity to do so in a person with AIDS.

What Is AIDS-Related Complex?

In AIDS-related complex (ARC), the patient tests positive for infection with HIV and has symptoms that are often less severe than those of AIDS. Signs and symptoms of ARC may include loss of appetite, weight loss, fever, night sweats, skin rashes, diarrhea, tiredness, lack of resistance to infection, and swollen lymph nodes. These are all signs and symptoms of many other diseases as well; only a physician can make an accurate diagnosis.

What Is HIV-Infected?

Some people remain apparently well for many years after infection with the AIDS virus. They may have no physically apparent symptoms of illness. However, they are able to spread the AIDS virus.

How Is the AIDS Virus Spread?

Blood, semen, and possibly vaginal secretions carry the AIDS virus. Most cases of AIDS have been spread by sexual contact or by sharing an intravenous drug needle with a person who has AIDS or who is infected with the virus. An infant whose mother or father is infected with the AIDS virus may be born with the infection or with AIDS. Although the occurrence is far less frequent, the virus can be spread to people who receive blood transfusions, transplanted organs or tissues, or donated sperm.

The virus is not spread by sharing food or towels, using swimming pools or hot tubs, sneezing, or using public toilets.

Who Is at High Risk for AIDS?

Drug Abusers

People who inject substances into their veins with shared needles make up to 25 percent of AIDS cases. The virus is spread by contaminated blood left in the needle, syringe, or other drug-related implements.

Demographics of AIDS Cases in the United States, September 1987

Adults

Homosexual/bisexual men	66%
Intravenous drug abusers	17%
Male homosexuals and intravenous drug abusers	8%
Hemophilia/coagulation disorders	1%
Heterosexual contact	4%
Transfusion-related AIDS	2%
Undetermined	3%

Children

Contracted AIDS from a parent	78%
Hemophilia/coagulation disorder	6%
Transfusion-related AIDS	12%
Undetermined	4%

Homosexual and Bisexual Men

Men who have sexual relations with other men are especially at risk. About 70 percent of AIDS victims throughout the country are male homosexuals and bisexuals. The U.S. Surgeon General has predicted that this percentage will probably decline as heterosexual transmission increases.

Children of AIDS Patients

Approximately two-thirds of pediatric AIDS cases are a result of transmission from an infected mother to her child. Most of these women are intravenous drug abusers or the sexual partners of intravenous drug abusers. It is expected that 65 percent of the infants born to infected women will develop AIDS.

People with Multiple Sex Partners

The risk of infection increases according to the number of sexual partners one has, male or female. The more partners, the greater the risk of becoming infected with the AIDS virus.

Patients with Hemophilia

Some people with this blood-clotting disorder have been infected with the AIDS virus either through a blood transfusion or by using blood products that help their blood to clot. This group represents a very small percentage of the cases of AIDS, and improved methods of testing and preparing blood and blood products have made this method of transmission unlikely in the future.

Blood Transfusion Recipients

All blood donors are screened to eliminate high-risk people. In addition, since March 1985, blood that has been collected for use has been tested for the presence of the AIDS virus.

What Is Safer Sex?

The U.S. Surgeon General recommends the following precautions to avoid either spreading or becoming infected by the AIDS virus during sexual relations:

- Anyone who has engaged in high-risk sexual activities or who has injected intravenous drugs into the body should have a blood test to determine if the AIDS virus is present.

- A person whose AIDS test is positive or who engages in high-risk activities and has not been tested should tell his or her sexual partner. If the decision is made to engage in sex despite the infection, a condom should be used. The use of condoms is recommended as a precautionary measure, since there is no other known effective barrier against HIV.

- A person whose partner has a positive AIDS test or who is suspected of having been exposed to the virus by previous heterosexual or homosexual behavior or through the use of intravenous drugs with shared needles or syringes should always use a condom during sex.

- A person who is at high risk for AIDS, or whose partner is at high risk, should avoid mouth contact with the penis, vagina, or rectum.

- People should avoid all sexual activities that could cause cuts or tears in the lining of the rectum, vagina, or penis.

● Sexual encounters with prostitutes should be avoided. Male and female prostitutes frequently are intravenous drug abusers and are at high risk of being infected with HIV.

How Many Americans Have AIDS?

The U.S. Public Health Service reports that between June 1981 and September 1987 nearly 42,000 Americans were diagnosed as having AIDS, and there have been over 24,000 deaths. The Centers for Disease Control have estimated that 1.5 million Americans are infected with the AIDS virus and predict that about 30 percent of these people, or almost 500,000, will develop AIDS within 4 years.

What Does AIDS Cost Our Country?

The total cost of medical care for AIDS patients in 1985 is estimated to have been $630 million, and in 1986, $1.1 billion. A report from the Health Economics Department, Palo Alto Medical Foundation/Research Institute, has predicted that medical care costs will rise to $8.5 billion by 1991. In 1985 this was 0.2 percent of all medical care expenditures for the U.S. population; by 1991 it is expected to be 1.4 percent.

Indirect costs of lost productivity due to illness and early death have been estimated at $3.9 billion in 1985; $7 billion in 1986, and $55.6 billion in 1991. These indirect costs were estimated to be 1.2 percent of the indirect costs of all illnesses in 1985 and 2.1 percent in 1986. By 1991 the indirect cost of AIDS is expected to be 12 percent of all indirect illness costs.

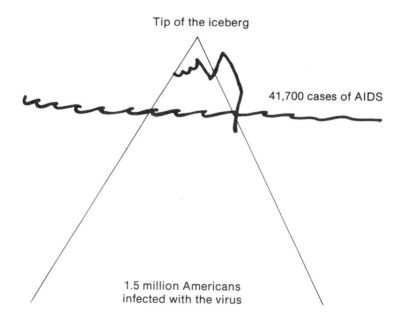

Tip of the iceberg

41,700 cases of AIDS

1.5 million Americans
infected with the virus

Projections for AIDS Cases - 1991, United States

Category	1986	1991
Cases diagnosed		
Cumulative cases at beginning of year	19,000	196,000
Diagnosed during year	16,000	74,000
Cumulative cases at end of year	35,000	270,000
Deaths		
Cumulative deaths at beginning of year	9,000	125,000
Deaths during year	9,000	54,000
Cumulative deaths at end of year	18,000	179,000

Source: Adapted from PHS Plan for Prevention and Control of AIDS and the AIDS virus; Public Health Reports, 101:341–348, 1986

How Much Money Is Being Spent on AIDS Research?

In 1986, the National Institutes of Health spent nearly $135 million on AIDS research; in 1987, the amount is expected to be over $252 million, and approximately $450 million will be spent in 1988.

What Have Researchers Learned about AIDS?

Researchers first identified the virus that was causing illness and death around the world and then learned how the disease was being spread.

Several different screening tests for AIDS infection have been developed. Testing is done both to learn if an individual has the virus and to determine if donated blood is contaminated with the AIDS virus.

Many different approaches to the development of AIDS vaccines are now being pursued by researchers, and plans to begin testing some vaccines for safety were announced in mid-1987. A variety of drugs thought to provide effective treatment for AIDS or for some of its opportunistic infections are being developed. Some have reached the stage of clinical trials. One medication, known as AZT, has been approved for treating some AIDS patients.

What Is the Outlook for AIDS?

The U.S. Surgeon General has stated that preventive behavior will protect the American public and contain the AIDS epidemic. Educational programs in the schools and in the workplace, by labor unions and health professionals, are needed so that Americans will learn how to avoid contracting AIDS and to protect those who have either the infection or the disease from unnecessary social isolation.

However, until the number of cases of AIDS declines, there will be a great need for inpatient and outpatient facilities to care for AIDS patients, along with home care programs and counseling and psychologic support services for both patients and family members. Programs to train chaplains, clergy, social workers, and volunteers to deal with AIDS and AIDS patients are needed.

Where Can One Obtain More Information on AIDS?

The free Public Health Service National AIDS hotline number is 1 (800) 342-AIDS.

National Institute of Allergy and Infectious Diseases
Office of Research Reporting and Public Response
Building 31, Room 7A32
Bethesda, MD 20892
(301) 496-5717

National Cancer Institute
Office of Cancer Communications
Building 31, Room 10A30
Bethesda, MD 20892
(301) 496-6631

Centers for Disease Control
1600 Clifton Road NE
Atlanta, GA 30333
(404) 329-3286

AIDS Action Council
729 Eighth St., S.E.
Suite 200
Washington, DC 20003
(202) 547-3101

Gay Men's Health Crisis
Box 274
132 W. 24th Street
New York, NY 10011
(212) 807-6664

AIDS Patient Care, a bimonthly magazine
for health care professionals
AIDS Research and Human Retroviruses
a bimonthly journal
and

*AmFAR Directory of Experimental Treatments
for AIDS & ARC*
Mary Ann Liebert, Inc., Publishers
1651 Third Avenue
New York, NY 10128
(212) 289-2300

For referral to local AIDS education and resource projects:

American Foundation for AIDS Research (AmFAR)
40 West 57th Street
New York, NY 10001
(212) 333-3118

For a free copy of the Surgeon General's Report on AIDS, write:

P.O. Box 14252
Washington, DC 20044

Glossary

Antibody. A protein produced in response to foreign material that enters the body
Cell-mediated immunity. The portion of the immune system mediated by small white
   blood cells called T cells or T lymphocytes
Hemophilia. A disorder of blood coagulation that may involve treatment with blood
   products
Human immunodeficiency virus (HIV). The virus responsible for causing AIDS
Immune reaction or response. The activity of various specialized body cells and chem-
   icals against foreign substances
Immune system. The complex system of cells and chemicals that reacts against foreign
   substances entering the body and fights off disease and infection
Immunity. The overall capability of an individual to resist or overcome an infection
Immunodeficiency. A condition that results from a defect in the immune system
Immunosuppression. A blunting of the immune response
Incubation period. The time between infection and the onset of symptoms
Kaposi's sarcoma. A type of cancer

Lymphocyte. A white blood cell important in immunity. There are two major types:
T lymphocytes processed by the thymus and involved in cell-mediated immunity;
B lymphocytes derived from the bone marrow and the precursors of the cells
(plasma cells) that produce antibody

Opportunistic infections. Illnesses caused by organisms that are not usually a threat
to people whose immune systems are functioning normally

Pneumocystis carinii *pneumonia* (PCP): A protozoan infection of the lungs

Serum. The yellow, liquid part of the blood remaining after cells and fibrin are removed

T cells. White blood cells processed in the thymus and responsible for cell-mediated
immunity

T lymphocytes. T cells

Sources

U.S. Surgeon General's Report on AIDS
National Institute of Allergy and Infectious Diseases
National Commission to Prevent Mortality
AIDS Action Council
National Commission to Prevent Infant Mortality

Alcoholism and Alcohol Abuse

What Is Alcoholism?

Alcoholism is loss of control over drinking alcoholic beverages. Alcoholics are people who experience symptoms of physical dependency on alcohol. Alcoholism has been described as mankind's most insidious disease. It is a complex, progressive disorder, typically creeping up on its victims over a period of 5 to 10 years of social drinking. It is a chronic, progressive, and potentially fatal disease, characterized by either tolerance to and physical dependency on alcohol, or pathologic organ changes, or both.

What Is Alcohol Abuse?

Alcohol abusers are people who are not physically dependent upon alcohol but who experience negative consequences as a result of its use. These consequences may include involvement in an accident or impairment of health or job performance.

Who Is Most Affected by Alcoholism?

The average alcoholic, according to the National Council on Alcoholism, is a person in their middle 30s with a good job. Chances are two to one that he or she began drinking in high school, and there is a 50 percent chance that one or both of the person's parents suffered from alcoholism. Only about 3 to 5 percent of alcoholics fit the down-and-out skid row stereotype.

How Many People Are Alcoholics or Have Alcohol-Related Problems?

An estimated 18 million Americans were said to be either alcohol abusers or alcoholics in 1985. Of this number, 10.6 million were alcoholics, those people who experience symptoms of alcohol dependence, and 7.3 million were alcohol abusers, who experience negative consequences of alcohol use (including arrest, involvement in an accident, impairment of health or job performance) but had not shown such signs of alcohol dependence as tolerance or withdrawal symptoms.

In 1985, an estimated 4.6 million adolescents, ages 14 to 17, experienced such negative consequences of alcohol use as poor school performance, trouble with parents, or involvement with law enforcement personnel. One of three American adults says that alcohol abuse has brought trouble to his or her family.

In 1986, 1.2 million people were treated at publicly funded alcohol treatment facilities, according to the National Association of State Alcoholism and Drug Abuse Program Directors.

How Many Americans Die from Alcohol-Related Problems?

In 1987, over 100,000 deaths are expected from alcohol-related causes, including deaths from cirrhosis and other direct medical consequences, alcohol-related motor vehicle accidents, and alcohol-related homicides, suicides, and nonmotor vehicle accidents. In addition, alcohol can contribute to other fatal illnesses, including cardiac myopathy, high blood pressure, pneumonia, and several types of cancer. Alcohol may also reduce the immune response to disease.

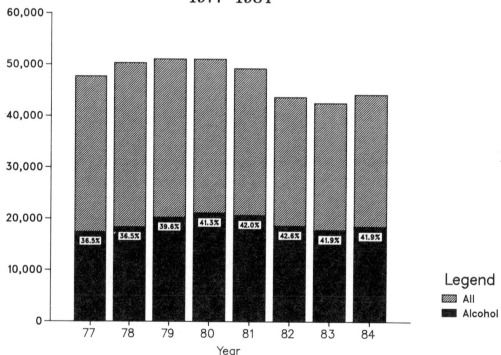

Proportion of Total Traffic Deaths Accounted for by Alcohol–Related Fatalities 1977–1984

Source: NIAAA. Surveillance Report No. 1

What Other Problems Does Alcohol Cause?

About 65 of 100 people in the United States will be in an alcohol-related traffic crash during their lifetime. At least 18,000 traffic deaths in the United States were alcohol-related in 1984. Alcohol is a contributing factor to at least 15,000 deaths and 6 million injuries in nonhighway accidents each year. It contributes to about 8,000 fatal and over 3 million nonfatal injuries in the home annually.

Fifty-four percent of jail inmates convicted of violent crimes were drinking before they committed the offense. Alcohol is involved in over 25 percent of marital violence cases, 33 percent of child molestation incidents, and 13 percent of child abuse cases.

What Is the Economic Cost to the Country of Alcoholism and Alcohol-Related Problems?

The cost of alcoholism and alcohol-related problems was $116.7 billion in 1983, and the annual cost has risen by at least another $20 billion since then. Of the figure cited for 1983, only $24.1 billion was for medical care; the indirect cost in lost earnings was $92.6 billion. The Congressional Office of Technology Assessment says that alcoholism and alcohol abuse may be responsible for up to 15 percent of the country's health care costs, which exceed $422 billion annually.

In 1986, $1.6 billion was spent for publicly funded alcohol and drug abuse treatment services. Three fourths of the people serviced by these facilities were treated for alcohol problems.

What Have Been the Most Significant Research Advances Relating to Alcohol Abuse and Alcoholism in the Past 10 Years?

Researchers have found that there are genetically transmitted determinants of alcoholism, and they have described varieties and stages of dependence. Tolerance to alcohol and physical dependence are now known not to be a single phenomenon. The knowledge that alcoholism results from a complex interplay of biologic and environmental factors has allowed the development of new approaches to prevention, intervention, and treatment programs, directed at current or potential alcohol abusers or alcoholics.

Raising the legal age for purchasing alcohol to 21 in most states, accomplished under pressure from the federal government, has reduced the number of alcohol-related automobile fatalities.

Recognition of the dangers and potential liabilty of serving alcohol to a person who appears to have had too much to drink also is seen as a way of reducing the toll of alcohol-caused accidents. Some states require commercial servers to be trained to recognize and deal with such problems.

How Much Money Is Being Spent on Research Relating to Alcoholism?

For fiscal year 1987, the National Institute on Alcohol Abuse and Alcoholism had a total research budget of $69 million.

What Is the General Outlook for Alcoholics?

Researchers are still learning about the organ damage produced by excessive intake of alcohol and its possible reversibility. Treatments for alcohol-induced organ damage are being studied.

Alcoholism treatment has become increasingly multimodal and multidisciplinary and may include support services and therapy for family members as well. Continual evaluation of new methods and attempts to match each patient to the most appropriate and effective type of treatment hold promise of improved and cost-effective results for the future.

Where Can One Obtain More Information on Alcoholism?

National Institute on Alcohol Abuse and Alcoholism
5600 Fishers Lane
Rockville, MD 20857
(301) 443-4883

Reference Desk
The National Clearinghouse for Alcohol and Drug Information
P.O. Box 2345
Rockville, MD 20852
(301) 468-2600

The National Council on Alcoholism, Inc.
12 West 21st Street
7th Floor
New York, NY 10010
(212) 206-6770

Alcoholics Anonymous
Box 459
Grand Central Station
New York, NY 10163
or for further information
look up Alcoholics Anonymous
in your local phone book

Glossary

Additives. The U.S. Bureau of Alcohol, Tobacco, and Firearms (BATF) permits the use of more than 30 chemicals in alcoholic beverages to stabilize, clarify, enhance color, improve taste, and aid fermentation; most are considered harmless, but some people, such as asthmatics, may be allergic to sulfite agents or other ingredients

Al-Anon family groups. A free self-help organization made up of friends and families of alcoholics; the groups are confidential, so the privacy of individual members is protected

Alateen. A self-help group of children of alcoholics

Alcohol. The active ingredient—the one that intoxicates—in beer, wine, and distilled spirits; ethyl alcohol or ethanol

Alcoholics Anonymous (AA). The largest self-help group for recovering alcoholics with more than a million members in 114 countries; there are chapters in almost all areas of the United States, and privacy of all members is assured

Blood alcohol concentration (BAC). Most state laws define intoxicated driving by a standard on a BAC scale. In many states, people who drive with a BAC level of 0.10 percent are legally guilty of driving while intoxicated (DWI), although driving is impaired at much lower levels. American Medical Association has recommended that the BAC level be lowered to 0.05 for DWI

Cirrhosis. A serious disease that occurs when scar tissue cuts off the liver's blood supply to the areas of the body responsible for making and storing nutrients; the most common cause of death in alcoholics

Delirium tremens (DTs). Serious withdrawal symptoms experienced by some, but not all, alcoholics when they stop drinking

Minimum legal drinking age. In most states, age 21

Proof. Standard measure of how much pure alcohol (ethyl alcohol) is in liquor; percentage of alcohol contained in a bottle can be determined by dividing the proof in half

Server responsibility. Some states have laws that hold those who serve alcoholic beverages legally responsible for accidents that may follow within a specified time

Sources

National Institute on Alcohol Abuse and Alcoholism
American Psychiatric Association
National Council on Alcoholism, Inc.

Alzheimer's Disease

What Is Alzheimer's Disease?

Alzheimer's disease is a progressive, irreversible, neurologic disorder. Symptoms include gradual memory loss, decline in ability to perform routine tasks, impairment of judgment, disorientation, personality change, difficulty in learning, and loss of language skills.

The physical changes most commonly associated with Alzheimer's disease occur in the proteins of the nerve cells in the cerebral cortex—the outer layer of the brain—leading to an accumulation of abnormal fibers called "neurofibrillary tangles" and degenerated nerve endings call "plaque." At first, the person with Alzheimer's disease will experience only minor symptoms that are often attributed to emotional upsets or other physical illnesses.

Gradually, the person becomes more forgetful, particularly about recent events. He or she may neglect to turn off the oven, misplace things, recheck to see if a task was done, take longer to complete a chore that was previously routine, or repeat already answered questions. As the disease progresses, memory loss increases and other changes, such as confusion, irritability, restlessness, and agitation, are likely to appear in personality, mood, and behavior. Judgment, concentration, orientation, and speech may also be affected. In the most severe stages, the disease renders its victims totally incapable of caring for themselves.

What Causes Alzheimer's Disease?

The cause of the disease is not known, but there may be a genetic predisposition to Alzheimer's disease or a not yet understood environmental factor.

Why Is Alzheimer's Disease Such a Problem?

Alzheimer's disease is a problem because of the number of people affected and the tremendous personal and family burden it creates. Sixty-six percent of all people with dementia are thought to have Alzheimer's disease. The majority of victims are among the population of aging Americans. As this group grows, so does the number of people with Alzheimer's disease. It is also a problem because Alzheimer's disease can strike people as young as age 45, at a time when they are usually in their most productive years and may be caring for a family.

There is no known cure for Alzheimer's disease, and families caring for a patient with the condition usually are under a tremendous strain. Often the patient is placed in a nursing home or other long-term care facility, at great expense to either the family or the government agency paying for the care.

How Many People Have Alzheimer's Disease? How Many Die?

The National Institute of Neurological and Communicative Disorders and Stroke estimates that there are 3 million Americans with Alzheimer's disease. Other estimates vary widely, and one researcher has estimated that 11 percent of the population over age 65 may have the disease. About half of all elderly people with severe intellectual impairment have Alzheimer's disease, according to the National Institute on Aging, and more than half the people in nursing homes in the U.S. have Alzheimer's disease.

The Alzheimer's Disease and Related Disorders Association states that more than 100,000 Americans die each year of Alzheimer's disease.

What Does Alzheimer's Disease Cost the Nation?

The National Institute of Neurological and Communicative Disorders and Stroke estimates that Alzheimer's disease cost Americans a total of $50 billion in health care expenditures and lost wages during 1986.

How Much Money Is Being Spent on Alzheimer's Disease Research?

In 1987, the National Institutes of Health allocated over $64 million for research related to Alzheimer's disease. This research is being carried out under the auspices of the National Institute of Neurological and Communicative Disorders and Stroke, National Institute on Aging, National Institute of Allergy and Infectious Diseases, and the Division of Research Resources.

What Progress Have Researchers Made in the Past 10 Years in Learning About Alzheimer's Disease?

A number of methods to diagnose Alzheimer's disease have been or are being developed. Psychologic tests are beginning to focus more closely on early signs of Alzheimer's disease, and researchers are learning to identify the disease through computed tomography (CT), magnetic resonance imaging (MRI), and positron emission tomography (PET) scans.

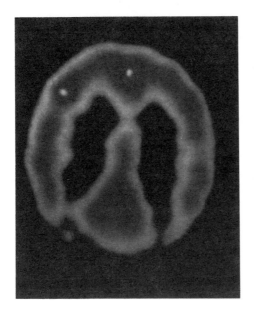
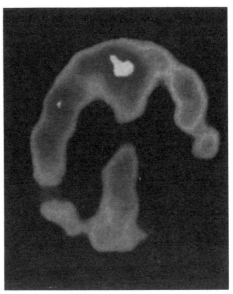

Normal Brain   Alzheimer's Disease Brain

PET scans showing dramatic differences in brain metabolism.
Source: NIH

Improved methods of diagnosis are important because there are other conditions—depression, multiinfarct dementia, emotional stress—that can appear to be Alzheimer's disease. Since these other conditions may be treatable, it is important that patients not be misclassified as having Alzheimer's disease.

Among the research avenues being explored are the disease's molecular pathology and the roles of toxins, infectious agents, heredity, and possible head injury.

In 1984, the National Institute on Aging was authorized by Congress to establish Alzheimer's Disease Research Centers in major medical centers across the country, 10 of which are now funded. These centers act as a network for sharing new ideas and research results. It is hoped that the long-term reward will be a way to treat and perhaps prevent Alzheimer's disease. In the short term, these centers provide opportunities for better care of patients.

What Is the Outlook for Alzheimer's Disease?

Because more people are living longer and the likelihood of developing Alzheimer's disease increases as one ages, the number of people with the condition undoubtedly will continue to grow. Better understanding of the needs of families who are caring for Alzheimer's patients and of the emotional and financial drains they experience is needed.

Where Can One Obtain More Information on Alzheimer's Disease?

National Institute on Aging
National Institutes of Health
Information Center
Building 31, Room 5C35
9000 Rockville Pike
Bethesda, MD 20892
(301) 496-1752

National Institute of Neurological and Communicative Disorders and Stroke
Office of Scientific and Health Reports
Building 31, Room 8A06
Bethesda, MD 20892
(301) 496-5924

Alzheimer's Disease and Related Disorders Association
70 East Lake Street
Chicago, IL 60601
(312) 853-3060

Hotline: A nationwide 24-hour hotline provides information and links families who need assistance with nearby Chapters and Affiliates. Those wanting help may call 1 (800) 621-0379; Illinois residents, call 1 (800) 572-6037.

Glossary

Alzheimer, Alois (1864–1915). German physician who studied the relationship of changes in the structure of the nervous system to disease and who first described the changes in the disease that carries his name

Biochemistry. The science that deals with the chemistry of living things

Computerized tomography (CT or CAT scan). A diagnostic technique using a computer and x-rays to obtain a highly detailed image of the section of the body being studied

Dementia. Impairment or loss of mental powers

Electroencephalography (EEG). Recording of the electric activities of the brain by means of wires placed on the scalp, useful in detecting tumors, epilepsy, and brain damage

Filament. A delicate fiber or thread of protein found in the brain cells

Immunology. A science that deals with the processes through which individuals are able to resist, or become sensitive to, a particular disease

Intellectual impairment. Diminished capacity to think or understand

Metabolic disorder. Disturbance in the physical and chemical processes by which chemical compounds in the body are produced, maintained, and transformed into energy

Nerve cell. A neuron, the basic unit of the nervous system consisting of a cell body and its threadlike extensions for receiving and transmitting impulses

Nerve ending. The fine branchlike endings of the extensions that carry impulses away from or toward the body of a nerve cell

Neurologic functioning. The normal activities of the nervous system

Sources

National Institute on Aging
Alzheimer's Disease and Related Disorders Association

Arthritis

What Is Arthritis?

Arthritis means inflammation of a joint and is a term that includes about 100 different diseases. The following are among the most commonly occurring varieties.

Rheumatic arthritis. This is an autoimmune disorder, characterized by chronic inflammation of the thin layer of tissue that lines a joint. Three fourths of the people with rheumatoid arthritis are women. The disease usually begins between ages 20 and 50 and affects 7 million Americans.

Osteoarthritis. This degenerative joint disease causes changes in the joint that create pain and limit movement and may stiffen or fuse the joint. Everyone who lives long enough will probably get osteoarthritis to some degree. There are 16 million Americans with osteoarthritis—1 of every 14 people—and two thirds of them are women.

Gout. Gout is caused by an accumulation of uric acid in the blood, which produces crystals that settle in joints and other tissues, causing irritation and inflammation. This form of arthritis is much more common in men than in women. Nearly 2 million Americans have gout.

Ankylosing spondylitis. This is a chronic inflammatory disease of the spine, also known as spinal arthritis. It is believed to be a genetic disorder of the immune system. The symptoms may be self-limited and stop after several years. One fifth of 1 percent of Americans have this disease, which usually affects white men between ages 16 and 35. Nearly 2.5 million Americans show some x-ray evidence of this disease.

Juvenile arthritis. There are several forms of juvenile arthritis, some of which are different from the kinds of arthritis found in adults. The condition may be mild or serious, and its effects can change from day to day, even from morning to afternoon. Affected children may experience skin rash, fever, inflammation of the eyes, slowed growth, swelling of lymph nodes, fatigue, and swelling and pain in the muscles and joints. There are 50,000 American children with juvenile arthritis.

Systemic lupus erythematosus. Better known as "lupus," this is an autoimmune disease in which the body's defense system causes cells to attack the lining of joints and other tissues. Severe cases of the disease can damage the skin, kidneys, blood vessels, brain, nervous system, heart, and other internal organs. Lupus is fatal in rare instances. The Lupus Foundation of America says that there are about 500,000 Americans with lupus, 90 percent of them women. The disease occurs more frequently among blacks, Hispanics, and certain Native American groups than among the general population. (For more information, see the chapter on lupus in this book.)

Scleroderma. This connective tissue disease is caused by the overproduction of the protein, collagen. It usually starts between ages 20 and 40. Some cases of the disease are mild; others may become life-threatening. There are 22,000 Americans with scleroderma, and two to three times as many women have the disease as men.

Other types of arthritis include infectious arthritis, bursitis and tendinitis, fibrositis, Reiter's syndrome, psoriatic arthritis, polymyalgia rheumatica, polymyositis, and dermatomyositis.

Who Is Most Likely to Have Arthritis?

The disease most commonly strikes people between the ages of 20 and 50 and is usually chronic, lasting for life. More than two thirds of the people with arthritis in the U.S. are women. Most people over age 60 have some degree of osteoarthritis.

What Causes Arthritis?

No one knows what causes arthritis, but the most promising answer lies in the three-way link among several forms of arthritis, heredity, and an infectious agent. Research has found that in such forms of arthritis as rheumatoid arthritis, lupus, and scleroderma, there are certain genetic markers that make a person more susceptible to developing the disease. Now scientists are studying what triggers those markers in some people but not in others. Much evidence points to viruses as the cause.

How Many People Have Arthritis?

In 1987, there were 37 million people with arthritis in the U.S. This is an increase from 31 million in 1976. Each year, a million Americans develop arthritis, one person every 33 seconds. One of every seven people has arthritis, and one in every three families is affected.

Arthritis is the nation's number one crippling disease.

What Is the Cost to the Country of Arthritis?

Arthritis costs Americans nearly $9 billion per year in lost wages and medical care, according to the Arthritis Foundation.

Arthritis accounts for 500 million days of restricted activity and 26 million days lost from work. It is a leading cause of industrial absenteeism and follows heart diseases as the second leading reason for disability payments.

In addition to necessary medical costs, the Arthritis Foundation states that there is more health fraud than exists for any other disease, with $1 billion spent on unproven arthritis remedies each year.

THE STORY OF INFLAMMATION

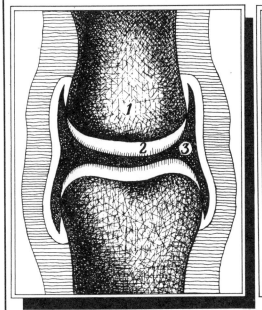

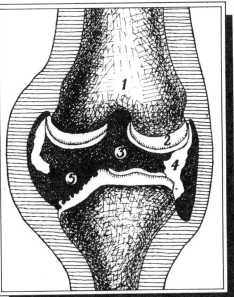

Normal Joint
1. Bone
2. Cartilage
3. Joint Fluid

Inflamed Joint
1. Bone
2. Cartilage
3. Joint Fluid
4. Thickened Synovial Lining
5. Pannus

■ Inflammation is what causes the swelling, redness, heat and pain of many kinds of arthritis. It causes or contributes to the damage inside joints and may lead to deformity and crippling. Inflammation in arthritis may be acute and self-limited or it may be chronic and persistent.

■ The inflammation of many types of arthritis is triggered by a foreign material. For example, a bacterial agent, as in infectious arthritis, a crystal in gout or pseudogout.

■ Inflammation is a *normal physiologic* response to a foreign invading material, whether it be bacterial, viral, crystalloid (such as uric acid crystals) or unknown.

■ In chronic persistent inflammation, such as is seen in rheumatoid arthritis, the body's normal defense system goes awry and cells programmed to defend become agents of destruction. (This is called autoimmunity.) This may result in further damage to the lining and cartilage of the joint.

■ In the inflammatory process, harmful substances, such as enzymes which attack and destroy cells of the joint lining and cartilage, may be released within the joint.

Source: Arthritis Foundation

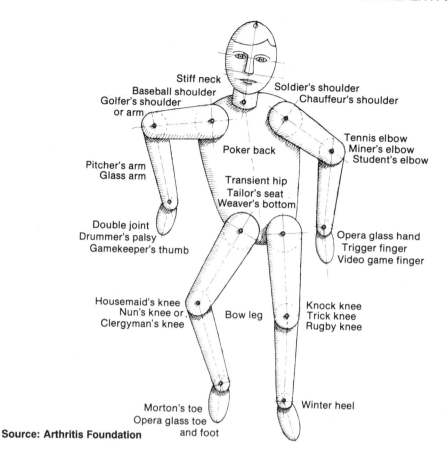

Source: Arthritis Foundation

How Much Money Is Spent for Arthritis Research?

The National Institutes of Health spent $104 million in 1986 and allocated an estimated $120 million in 1987. This money provided support for programs in the National Institute of Arthritis and Musculoskeletal and Skin Diseases, National Institute of Dental Research, National Institute of Diabetes and Digestive and Kidney Diseases, National Institute of Neurological and Communicative Diseases and Stroke, National Institute of Allergy and Infectious Diseases, National Institute of General Medical Sciences, National Institute of Child Health and Human Development, National Institute on Aging, and the Division of Research Resources.

The Arthritis Foundation spent $4.9 million on research during 1986.

What Progress Has Been Made in Arthritis Research in the Past 10 Years?

Major advances have taken place in the development of drugs to treat arthritis in recent years, increasing the available variety of analgesics (pain relievers), anti-inflammatories, and other medications.

Joint replacement surgery is highly effective for many patients; 100,000 hip replacements are performed in the U.S. every year. New surgical techniques and new materials for the replacement joints are among the benefits produced by recent research. In addition, new techniques of physical therapy, along with an improved understanding of appropriate exercise techniques, are enabling some people who have arthritis to function more fully.

What Is the Outlook for Arthritis Patients?

Researchers are continuing to try to understand better the diseases that cause arthritis. Until a way to prevent or cure the diseases is discovered, scientists will seek better medications and other techniques for relieving the discomfort caused by arthritis.

Among the major areas being investigated by arthritis researchers today are the cells' genetic markers, the body's immune system, and bacteria and viruses that may be infectious triggers of the disease. Medical scientists also are evaluating the possibilty of replacing worn cartilage, in the way that joints are now replaced.

Where Can One Obtain More Information on Arthritis?

National Institute of Arthritis and Musculoskeletal and Skin Diseases
Building 31, Room B2B15
Bethesda, MD 20892
(301) 496-8188

National Arthritis and Musculoskeletal and Skin Diseases
Information Clearinghouse
Box AMS
Bethesda, MD 20892
(301) 468-3235

Arthritis Foundation
1314 Spring Street, N.W.
Atlanta, GA 30309
(404) 872-7100

Glossary

Cartilage. Rubbery material that cushions the ends of the bones and absorbs shock
Fibrositis. A condition in which there is generalized pain in the muscles, ligaments, and tendons

Flare. A period during which disease symptoms reappear or become worse

Genetic marker. A specific tissue type, similar to a blood type, that is passed on from one generation to the next in the genes; some genetic markers are linked with certain rheumatic diseases

Gout. A form of arthritis in which the body builds up too much uric acid, crystals of which then collect in joints and cause painful attacks

Infectious arthritis. Arthritis that develops as a complication of an infection by a virus, bacterium, or fungus

Inflammation. Reaction of the body to injury or disease, causing pain, swelling, redness, warmth, and often reduced range of motion in the affected area

Joint. Any place in the body where two bones articulate

Ligament. A strong cordlike structure that connects bones to other bones

Physiatrist. A medical doctor specializing in physical medicine and rehabilitation

Remission. A period during which disease symptoms are reduced or absent

Rheumatic diseases. A group of diseases that affect muscles, ligaments, tendons, joints, and sometimes other body parts, e.g., the heart

Rheumatologist. A medical doctor specializing in diagnosis and treatment of arthritis or other rheumatic diseases

Systemic disease. One that can affect many parts of the body, not only a small area

Tendinitis. Inflammation of a tendon

Tendon. The strong, cordlike, tapered end of a muscle that connects the muscle to a bone

Uric acid. A chemical in the body that, in gout, changes into crystals and collects in joints, causing painful attacks

Sources

Arthritis Foundation
National Institute of Arthritis and Musculoskeletal and Skin Diseases

Asthma

What Is Asthma?

Asthma is a disease that usually occurs in episodes or attacks. The air tubes of the lungs are narrowed by tightened muscles, mucous plugs, and swollen tissues. The person then has trouble breathing. The episodes may come on suddenly, or they may develop slowly over hours or days. They may last only a few minutes or go on for a few hours.

People with asthma are said to have sensitive lung tissues, which react more than they should to such stimuli as an allergen or irritant, cold air, a viral infection, vigorous exercise, or a combination of these and other factors. Excitement and emotion may contribute to an attack, says the American Lung Association, but the disease is a physical, not a psychologic, disorder.

How Many People Have Asthma? How Many Deaths Does It Cause?

Nearly 9 million people in the United States have asthma, according to 1986 estimates. More than 2 million of these asthmatics are under 17 years of age, and half of the people who now have asthma developed the disease before they were 18. A recent study found a higher than expected number of adults who developed asthma after the age of 60.

In 1985, 3,760 Americans died from asthma, a number that has been slowly rising over the past decade. The American Academy of Allergy and Immunology states that asthma may also have been a contributing cause of another 16,000 deaths. Increases in asthma deaths have occurred in the U.S. and in Australia, Denmark, Canada, and England.

What Is the Economic Cost of Asthma to the Country?

Asthma is estimated to have cost Americans nearly $3.9 billion in 1986. This includes more than $2.5 billion per year for medical care and over $1.3 billion in such indirect costs as time lost from work.

Asthma was recorded as responsible for 462,000 separate hospital stays during 1985, and it was responsible for an estimated 35 million days spent in bed.

Trend in Deaths From Asthma
U.S., 1968 to 1985

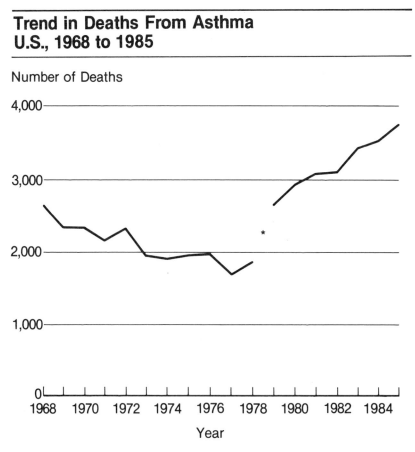

Number of Deaths

* Break in Comparability Due to Revision of the International Classification of Diseases.

Source: Vital Statistics of the U.S., National Center for Health Statistics

How Much Money Is Spent for Research on Asthma?

In 1986, the National Institutes of Health spent about $15 million on asthma research; in 1987, it allocated an estimated $17 million.

What Progress Has Been Made in Research on Asthma during the Past 10 Years?

There is no drug that cures asthma, but there are drugs that can relieve symptoms, and new medications are helping people with asthma and increasing the number of ways they can control their disease.

Educational efforts by voluntary health agencies and the National Heart, Lung, and Blood Institute are reaching out to children with asthma and their families to help them to understand this chronic disease. Materials to help teach children and adults how to help control the disease have been developed in recent years. Improved methods of identifying and controlling allergies are also helpful to many people with asthma.

What Is the Outlook for People with Asthma?

Researchers are concerned about the increasing number of deaths from asthma after many years of decline and are seeking to find a cause. The hopeful news is that the National Institute of Allergy and Infectious Diseases reports that 98 percent of people with asthma are able to control their disease effectively through medication and other treatments.

Where Can One Obtain More Information on Asthma?

National Institute of Allergy and Infectious Diseases
Office of Communications
Building 31, Room 7A32
Bethesda, MD 20892
(301) 496-5717

National Heart, Lung, and Blood Institute
National Institutes of Health
Office of Prevention, Education and Control
Building 31, Room 4A21
Bethesda, MD 20892
(301) 496-4236

American Lung Association
1740 Broadway
New York, NY 10019-4374
(212) 315-8700

American Academy of Allergy and Immunology
611 East Wells Street
Milwaukee, WI 53202
(414) 272-6071

Joint Council of Allergy and Immunology
800 East Northwest Highway
Palatine, IL 60067
(312) 359-3090

Glossary

Airway obstruction. A narrowing, clogging, or blocking of the airways that carry air to the lungs; a major problem in an acute asthmatic attack

Allergen. A substance capable of causing an allergic reaction, e.g., plant pollens, mold spores, and animal danders

Allergic reaction. An adverse immune response following contact with otherwise harmless substances, such as pollens, molds, foods, cosmetics, and drugs

Allergy. An altered immune response to a specific substance, such as ragweed pollen, on reexposure to it

Alveoli. The lung's tiny air sacs

Antigen. Any substance that provokes an immune response when introduced into the body

Antihistamine. A drug that blocks the effects of histamine, a chemical responsible for many of the symptoms of allergy when released by the body's mast cells during an allergic reaction

Bronchi. The tubes that branch from the windpipe, one to each lung, through which air enters and leaves the lungs

Challenge test. A medical procedure used to identify the substances to which a person is sensitive by deliberate exposure to dilute amounts until allergic symptoms are provoked

Elimination diet. A restricted diet in which foods suspected of causing allergic reactions are eliminated from the diet, and then reintroduced one at a time so that the allergens can be identified

Immunotherapy. Injections of gradually increasing amounts of allergens known to trigger a patient's allergic response; also called desensitization, hyposensitization, injection therapy, and allergy shots

Patch tests. A form of skin testing in which suspected allergens are applied to the skin, covered, and observed for several days to see if a reaction occurs

Provocative test. Challenge test

Radioallergosorbent test (RAST). A test for measuring the amount of specific antibodies in a patient's blood to help identify allergens

Sensitize. Immunize; to administer or expose to an antigen provoking an immune response so that, on later exposure to that antigen, a more vigorous secondary response will occur

Skin tests. Injection of a small, dilute amount of allergen under the skin or application to a scratch on the patient's arm or back; if the patient is allergic to that substance, a small raised area surrounded by redness will appear at the test site within 15 minutes

Spirometer. A device that measures the amount of air inhaled and exhaled. The amount of airway obstruction in patients also can be calculated

Sources

National Institute of Allergy and Infectious Diseases
American Lung Association
American Academy of Allergy and Immunology

Blindness and Visual Impairment

What Are Blindness and Visual Impairment?

Blindness is total or virtually total loss of vision. People who are legally blind may have some amount of useful vision and are among those who may be described as severely visually impaired. People who have a diagnosed vision problem that is not correctable but is not disabling are said to be visually impaired (but not severely impaired); this includes people who are blind in one eye or color deficient or who have glaucoma or cataracts that have not affected their vision severely.

Most eye diseases and the visual disability they cause do not affect other parts of the body. However, diabetes and several other systemic diseases can simultaneously affect the eye and other organs. Aging is also a factor common to many eye diseases and other disorders affecting health. Thus, the visually impaired person often has other health problems in addition to eye disease.

What Causes Blindness and Visual Impairment?

Glaucoma. This condition is caused by the presence of too much fluid in the eye. When untreated, glaucoma causes the loss of central and side vision. It is the single leading cause of blindness in the U.S., accounting for 13 percent of all blindness and 12 percent of all new cases. Early detection and treatment with the proper medication can prevent blindness from this disease.

Macular degeneration. The degeneration of the central part of the retina is the leading cause of blindness in the elderly and the second leading cause of blindness among people of all ages. It accounts for 17 percent of all new blindness and causes at least some loss of vision in 10 million people over the age of 50.

Cataract. This clouding of the eye's lens is the third leading cause of blindness in the U.S., accounting for 8 percent of all blindness and 10 percent of all new cases. The vast majority of people whose cataracts are treated surgically regain their vision with the aid of implants, glasses, or contact lenses. More than a million cataract surgeries are performed in the U.S. each year.

Diabetic retinopathy. This is the most frequent eye complication of diabetes. It is the fourth leading cause of blindness in the general population and the leading cause of new blindness among people ages 20 to 74. Laser surgery can sometimes help to restore vision.

Retinitis pigmentosa. This inherited disease gradually destroys night vision and reduces peripheral vision. It is the fifth leading cause of blindness and accounts for 3 percent of all new cases of blindness.

Retrolental fibroplasia. This condition is caused by high oxygen levels in incubators during the first 10 days of life. It is a major cause of blindness among adults aged 20 to 44 because of an earlier lack of knowledge of its cause.

Retinal detachment. This condition occurs most often in men, the extremely near-sighted, and the aged and can occur as a result of a blow on the head. It can be due to tears or holes in the retina, extra fluid from an infection, blood vessel disturbance, or tumors. When early diagnosis of the problem is made, about 89 percent of detached retinas can be surgically reattached, restoring partial vision.

Injuries. About 4 percent of all blindness in the U.S. is caused by injuries, with nearly half of them happening in the home. Many experts believe that the use of proper eye safety equipment would prevent a large number of injuries.

Infant eye problems. A mother's infection during pregnancy can cause blindness in an infant. The causes can include syphilis, gonorrhea, toxoplasmosis, rubella, and other viral infections.

Corneal diseases. Although diseases of the cornea account for only about 6 percent of legal blindness in the U.S., they are the primary cause of blindness worldwide. They are also the most painful of all eye disorders and account for considerable disability.

How Many People Are Visually Impaired?

The National Eye Institute estimates that 1.7 million Americans have a visual impairment that is both severe and irreversible. There are 11 million people in the U.S. who are considered nonseverely visually impaired.

About 500,000 Americans are legally blind, and 8 percent of this group is under age 20. Over 3 million people in the U.S. are blind in one eye; in about 2 percent of these cases, the other eye is defective but not blind.

It has been estimated that 47,000 Americans lose their sight each year—one person every 11 minutes.

What Is the Cost of Visual Impairment to This Country?

Blindness costs this country over $20 billion per year in direct and indirect costs.

How Much Money Is Spent on Vision-Related Research Each Year?

The National Eye Institute allocated nearly $217 million for research in 1987.

What Has Research Contributed to the Prevention and Treatment of Visual Impairment in the Past 10 Years?

Lasers have been found effective in the treatment of diabetic retinopathy, age-related macular degeneration, glaucoma, and ocular histoplasmosis.

Improved methods for corneal transplantation, as well as preservation of corneal tissue to be used in transplants, have been developed.

Even when a visual impairment cannot be corrected by medical or surgical means, there are many aids and services that can help the person to make the best use of his or her remaining vision. These aids and services include talking books, large-print reading matter, and various mobility aids. New devices are continually being developed, ranging from sophisticated machines, such as home computers for the visually impaired, to simple household items designed to make daily life easier.

Thanks to the research advances of the last decade, many common blinding diseases can be detected earlier and treated more effectively than ever before. There is even hope that in the future some eye diseases will be prevented altogether.

What Is the Outlook for People Who Are Blind or Visually Impaired?

Advocates for the blind and visually impaired are concerned that the cost of low vision aids, which can help many people function better, frequently is not covered by health insurance. In some states, Medicaid will pay for some of the needs of medically needy low vision patients, but Medicare does not cover low vision services for the elderly.

For those whose visual problems are caused by corneal disease, cataract, clouding of the clear gel (vitreous) that fills the middle of the eye, or recent detachment of the retina, modern surgical techniques offer good prospects for restoration of sight. For people whose impairment is caused by infection of the eye or inflammation of its inner tissues, there is a good chance that antibiotics or other medications can restore a considerable degree of visual function. These procedures and drugs are continually being improved through research, so those who develop such eye conditions in future years should have an even better chance of successful treatment.

However, if visual impairment is the result of serious damage to the retina, the optic nerve, or the part of the brain involved in sight, the vision that has been lost cannot be restored by any techniques known today. This is because no nerve tissue in the body can regenerate. The problem of nerve regeneration is under study, but it will be a long time before this research yields even an experimental method of restoring damaged nerve tissue in the visual system.

Where Can One Obtain More Information on Blindness?

National Eye Institute
Section of Scientific Reporting
National Institutes of Health
Building 31, Room 6A32
Bethesda, MD 20892
(301) 496-5248

American Academy of Ophthalmology
1101 Vermont Avenue, N.W.
Washington, DC 20005
(202) 737-6662

American Foundation for the Blind
15 West 16th Street
New York, NY 10011
(212) 620-2000

National Society to Prevent Blindness
500 E. Remington Road
Schaumburg, IL 60173
(312) 843-2020

Eye Bank Association of America, Inc.
1511 K Street, NW Suite 830
Washington, DC 20005-1401
(202) 628-4280

Eye Research Institute of Retina Foundation
20 Staniford Street
Boston, MA 02114
(617) 742-3140

Glossary

Age-related macular degeneration. Irreversible and progressive damage to the macular area of the retina, resulting in a gradual loss of fine or reading vision
Cataract. A clouding of the normally clear lens of the eye that interferes with vision; age-related (or senile) cataract is the most common type; congenital cataracts develop early in life

Cornea. Transparent covering at the front of the eye that is part of the eye's focusing system

Corneal transplantation. Surgery to transplant healthy donor corneal tissue into the eye of a person whose own cornea is diseased

Diabetic retinopathy. A complication of diabetes caused by deterioration of the small blood vessels that nourish the retina

Epikeratophakia. Surgery in which a very small piece of donor corneal tissue is placed on the recipient's cornea to change its curvature and focusing power

Glaucoma. Increased fluid pressure inside the eye that causes damage to the optic nerve and impairment of vision

Intraocular lens implant (IOL). A plastic lens inserted in the eye as a replacement for the natural lens removed during cataract surgery

Laser. An instrument that focuses an intense beam of light on a small area of living tissue; used by ophthalmologists to treat many eye diseases

Legal blindness. The definition of blindness used by states and the federal government; consists of (1) central visual acuity of 20/200 or poorer in the better eye, even with appropriate corrective lenses, or (2) a visual acuity better than 20/200 but a field of vision no greater than 20 degrees in its widest diameter

Lens. Transparent tissue behind the iris that focuses light rays on the retina

Low vision. Visual impairment that is sufficient to cause some limitation of a person's daily activities, even when corrected as much as possible, but not so severe that all useful vision is lost

Optic nerve. The nerve at the back of the eye that carries visual impulses from the retina to the brain

Retina. Light-sensitive tissue at the back of the eye that sends visual impulses by way of the optic nerve to the brain

Retinal detachment. Separation of the inner layer of the retina from the outer layer. This should be surgically repaired promptly

Senile macular degeneration. Age-related macular degeneration

Vitreous hemorrhage. Leakage of blood into the clear gel (vitreous) that fills the center of the eye

Sources

National Eye Institute
American Optometric Association
American Foundation for the Blind

Cancer

What Is Cancer?

Cancer is a large group of diseases characterized by uncontrolled growth and spread of abnormal cells. The tumor these cells create can invade and destroy surrounding normal tissue, and the disease, if not controlled, can cause death.

When cancer cells remain at their original site, the disease is said to be localized. If not diagnosed and treated, the cells may invade other organs or tissue, either by direct growth of the tumor or by being carried through the lymph or blood systems to other parts of the body. This is called metastasis.

What Causes Cancer?

Tobacco. Cigarette smoking is the single major cause of cancer deaths in the United States. Smokers have twice the cancer death rate as nonsmokers, and heavy smokers have more than a threefold greater risk. Smoking is responsible for 83 percent of lung cancer and 30 percent of all cancer deaths. Exposure to second-hand smoke increases the chances of developing lung cancer even in a nonsmoker. The use of smokeless tobacco increases the risk for cancers of the mouth, larynx, throat, and esophagus.

Diet. Obese people are at increased risk for colon, breast, and uterine cancers. A high-fat diet may be associated with breast, colon, and prostate cancers. High-fiber foods may help reduce the risk of colon cancer. Foods containing vitamins A and C may help lower the risk of cancers of the larynx, esophagus, stomach, and lung. Salt-cured, smoked, and nitrite-cured foods have been associated with esophageal and stomach cancers. Some experts have said that diet may be related to as much as 35 percent of all cancer deaths.

Sunlight. Almost all of the more than 500,000 cases of nonmelanoma skin cancer diagnosed each year in the U.S. are considered to be sun-related. Sun exposure also is thought to be a major factor in the development of melanoma.

Alcohol. Heavy drinkers of alcohol increase their likelihood of developing oral cancer and cancers of the larynx, throat, esophagus, and liver.

Estrogen. The use of estrogen by menopausal women should be discussed carefully by the woman and her physician in relation to benefits and risks.

Radiation. Excessive exposure to radiation can increase the risk of developing cancer.

Cancer Risk Factors

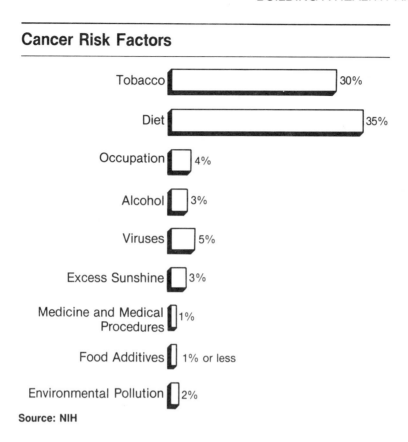

Tobacco 30%
Diet 35%
Occupation 4%
Alcohol 3%
Viruses 5%
Excess Sunshine 3%
Medicine and Medical Procedures 1%
Food Additives 1% or less
Environmental Pollution 2%

Source: NIH

Occupational hazards. Exposure to many industrial agents, which the American Cancer Society says include nickel, chromate, asbestos, and vinyl chloride, can increase the risk of cancer. Smokers who are exposed to these substances multiply their risks.

Air and water pollution. Although the National Cancer Institute has stated that evidence of the effects of pollution as a cause of cancer is not conclusive, it has been estimated that these factors may account for up to 5 percent of all cancers.

What Are the Major Cancer Sites?

Lung Cancer

Incidence. An estimated 150,000 new cases of lung cancer were diagnosed during 1987.

Mortality. About 136,000 people will die from lung cancer in 1987. The age-standardized lung cancer death rate for women is higher than that for any other cancer, even breast cancer.

Risk factors. Smoking cigarettes for 20 years or more is strongly associated with lung cancer, as is exposure to such industrial substances as asbestos, particularly in combination with smoking. Evidence now points to second-hand smoke as a cause of lung cancer; exposure to radiation is another risk factor.

Survival. Only 13 percent of lung cancer patients live 5 or more years after diagnosis. The rate is 33 percent for cases detected in a localized stage, but only 24 percent of lung cancers are discovered that early.

Colon and Rectal Cancer

Incidence. There was an estimate of 145,000 new cases in 1987, including 102,000 of colon cancer and 43,000 of rectal cancer. Their combined incidence is second only to that of lung cancer (excluding common skin cancers).

Mortality. There will be an estimated 60,000 deaths in 1987, second only to lung cancer. This includes 52,000 for colon cancer and 8,200 for rectal cancer.

Risk factors. Risk factors include personal or family history of colon and rectal cancer, personal or family history of polyps in the colon or rectum, and inflammatory bowel disease. Evidence suggests that bowel cancer may be linked to a diet high in fat or deficient in fiber.

Survival. The American Cancer Society states than when colorectal cancer is detected and treated in an early, localized stage, the 5-year survival rate is 86 percent for colon cancer, compared with 39 percent if it has spread to other parts of the body. For rectal cancer, the 5-year survival rate is 77 percent if the disease is localized and 31 percent if it has spread.

Breast Cancer

Incidence. There will be an estimated 130,000 new cases in the United States during 1987. About 1 of 10 women can be expected to develop breast cancer at some time during her life.

Mortality. The estimated 41,300 deaths (41,000 females, 300 males) in 1987 is second only in females to deaths from lung cancer, which is now the foremost cause of cancer deaths in women.

Risk factors. These include age over 50, personal or family history of breast cancer, never had children, and first child after age 30.

Survival. The 5-year survival rate for localized breast cancer has risen from 78 percent in the 1940s to 90 percent today. If the breast cancer has not spread, the survival rate approaches 100 percent. If the cancer has spread, the rate is 60 percent.

Skin Cancer

Incidence. The incidence is over 500,000 cases a year. The most serious skin cancer is malignant melanoma, which strikes about 26,000 men and women each year.

Mortality. There are an estimated 7,800 deaths a year (5,800 from malignant melanoma).

Risk factors. Risk factors include excessive exposure to the sun, fair complexion, occupational exposure to coal, tar, pitch, creosote, arsenic compounds, or radium. One study found that severe sunburn in childhood increases the risk of melanoma in later life.

Survival. The 5-year survival rate for white patients with malignant melanoma is 80 percent, compared with 95 percent for patients with other kinds of skin cancer. The 5-year survival rate for localized malignant melanoma is 89 percent; however, the survival rate once the disease has spread is reduced to 46 percent.

Uterine Cancer

Incidence. An estimated 48,000 new invasive cases will be found during 1987, including 13,000 cases of cervical cancer and 35,000 cases of cancer of the endometrium, or inner lining of the uterus. The incidence of invasive cervical cancer has decreased in recent years, whereas cancer in situ (localized and confined to one place; a very early stage) has risen in all groups. Cervical cancer is most common today in low socioeconomic groups, but all groups are at risk. Endometrial cancer is found mostly in women between the ages of 55 and 69.

Mortality. There will be an estimated 6,800 deaths in 1987 from cervical cancer and 2,900 from endometrial cancer. Overall, the death rate from uterine cancer has decreased more than 70 percent during the last 40 years, due mainly to use of the Pap test and regular checkups.

Risk factors. For cervical cancer, risk factors include early age at first intercourse and multiple sex partners. For endometrial cancer, risk factors include history of infertility, failure of ovulation, prolonged estrogen therapy, and obesity.

Survival rate. There has been a moderate improvement in survival rates for both uterine cancer sites during a recent 10-year period. The 5-year survival rate for cervical cancer patients, whites and blacks, is 66 percent. For patients diagnosed early, however, the rate is 80 to 90 percent. Cancer in situ has virtually a 100 percent survival rate. The figures for endometrial cancer are 83 percent in all stages, 91 percent for early cancers, and virtually 100 percent for endometrial precancerous lesions.

Leukemia

Incidence. There will be an estimated 26,400 new cases in 1987, about half of them acute leukemia and half of them chronic leukemia. Although it is often considered primarily a childhood disease, leukemia strikes many more adults (24,600 cases per year compared with 2,000 in children).

Mortality. There will be an estimated 17,800 deaths in 1987.

Risk factors. Leukemia, a cancer of the blood-forming tissues, strikes both sexes and all ages. Causes of most cases are unknown. A higher than normal incidence of

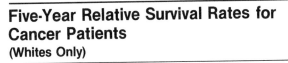

Five-Year Relative Survival Rates for Cancer Patients
(Whites Only)

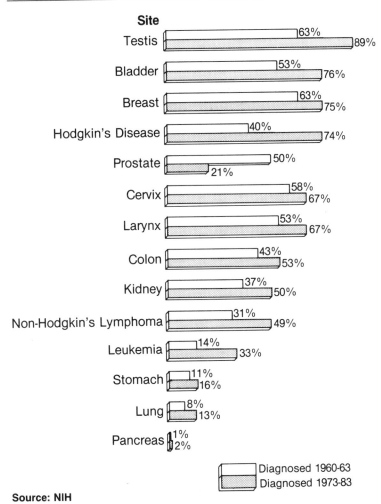

Site

Testis	63% / 89%
Bladder	53% / 76%
Breast	63% / 75%
Hodgkin's Disease	40% / 74%
Prostate	50% / 21%
Cervix	58% / 67%
Larynx	53% / 67%
Colon	43% / 53%
Kidney	37% / 50%
Non-Hodgkin's Lymphoma	31% / 49%
Leukemia	14% / 33%
Stomach	11% / 16%
Lung	8% / 13%
Pancreas	1% / 2%

Diagnosed 1960-63
Diagnosed 1973-83

Source: NIH

leukemia occurs in people with Down's syndrome and certain other hereditary conditions. It has been linked also to excessive exposure to radiation and certain chemicals, including benzene.

Survival. The average 5-year survival rate for white patients with leukemia is 33 percent, due partly to the very poor survival rate of patients with certain types of the disease, including acute granulocytic leukemia. The 5-year survival rate for blacks is 28 percent. Over the past 30 years, there has been an improvement in survival of patients with acute lymphocytic leukemia. In the early 1960s, the chances of surviving were only 4 percent; white males with the disease now have a 42 percent survival rate, white females a 49 percent survival rate, and white children a 68 percent survival rate. The American Cancer Society states that in some medical centers, optimum treatment has raised the survival rate of children with acute lymphocytic leukemia to 75 percent.

How Many Americans Get Cancer Each Year? How Many Die?

It is estimated that in 1987, about 965,000 people will be diagnosed as having cancer. This figure does not include the additional 500,000 Americans who are found to have nonmelanoma skin cancer each year. About 745 million Americans, or 30 percent of people now living, will eventually have cancer. The disease will strike in three of four families.

In 1986, an estimated 472,000 Americans died of cancer. In 1987, the disease is expected to take 483,000 lives, or one American every 65 seconds.

Despite the many advances in the detection and treatment of cancer, there has been a steady increase in the age-adjusted death rate. In 1935, the rate was 152 per 100,000 population; in 1984, it was 171. Lung cancer is blamed for this continuing increase. In 1935, lung cancer occurred in 6.1 per 100,000 population; in 1984, it was 45.6 per 100,000. Death rates from cancer at other major sites have been leveling off and even, in some cases, declining.

How Many People Alive Today Have Had Cancer?

There are over 5 million Americans alive today who have a history of cancer, 3 million of whom were diagnosed 5 or more years ago. Most of these 3 million can be considered cured, whereas others still have evidence of cancer. "Cured" means that a patient has no evidence of disease for the 5 years after treatment and has the same life expectancy as a person who never had cancer.

How Has the Survival Rate Changed Over the Past 50 Years?

In the 1930s, 20 percent of patients survived at least 5 years after treatment. In the 1940s, it was 25 percent, and in the 1960s, it was 33 percent. Today, 40 percent of patients who have cancer will be alive 5 years after diagnosis.

How Could the National Survival Rate Be Increased?

The national survival rate could be increased by at least 10 to 15 percent if every cancer patient received today's state-of-the-art treatment. An additional 170,000 people with cancer could probably have been saved by earlier diagnosis and treatment,

How cancer works

1. A carcinogen is a cancer-causing compound. It can be inhaled, enter the body through food and water, and in some cases be absorbed through the skin.

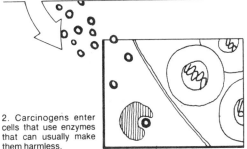

2. Carcinogens enter cells that use enzymes that can usually make them harmless.

2A. These detoxified chemicals — a vast majority — are excreted from the body. In this way, the body protects cells from damage.

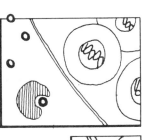

3. On rare occasions, the enzymes fail to detoxify and the carcinogens become more potent, gaining ability to bind to and damage genetic material within cells.

4. If the compound binds in the right place in the genetic material (DNA), it can cause abnormal growth when the cell divides.

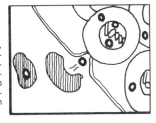

5. Normally a repair mechanism clips out the area with the carcinogen; repairs damage. If not, an abnormal gene is passed on.

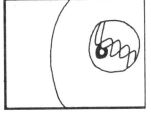

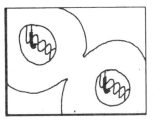

6. The abnormal gene can be a cancer gene or oncogene. But more than one such gene is needed. Before a tumor forms, one or more similar steps must occur. Some chemicals, called promotors, can speed this process if they reach the already damaged cells.

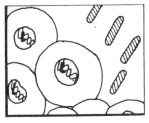

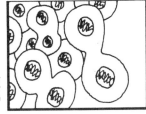

7. If there are two or more working cancer genes, they can spawn tumor formation.

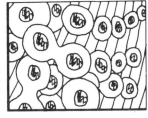

8. With the right genes, the cancer cells will have special enzymes that allow them to spread into the bloodstream.

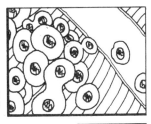

9. Malignant cells drift in bloodstream as far as they can.

9A. If the body recognizes the tumor cell in the blood stream as an "invader", the immune system attacks it. The body may send out white cells to engulf and destroy the cancer cell.

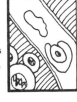

10. If tumor cell evades imune system, it will find a new home; resume growth, seeding new tumors.

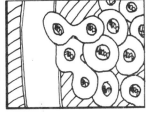

Source: American Association For The Advancement of Science

Source: The Sacramento Bee, September 15–October 3, 1985

CANCER INCIDENCE AND DEATHS BY SITE AND SEX—1987 ESTIMATES

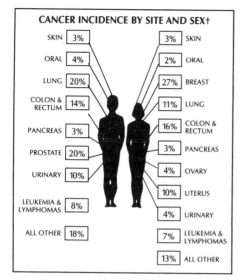

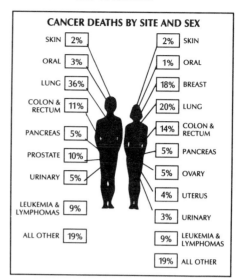

†Excluding non-melanoma skin cancer and carcinoma in situ.

Source: Cancer Facts and Figures—1987. American Cancer Society

according to the American Cancer Society. Such measures as examination by a physician for early colon and rectal cancer, Pap tests, and a combination of breast self-examination and mammography can help to diagnose a precursor of cancer or the disease in its early stages.

What Is the Total Cost to the Nation of Cancer?

Cancer cost the U.S. approximately $71.6 billion in 1985, according to the American Cancer Society. Of this amount, $21.8 billion was for medical care, $8.6 billion was for the cost of lost productivity, and $41.2 billion was the dollar amount put on the loss of productivity due to premature death.

Cancer accounts for 10 percent of the total cost of disease in the U.S.

How Much Money Is Being Spent on Cancer Research in the United States?

In 1987, the National Cancer Institute budgeted about $1.4 billion for cancer research, and additional money was spent on cancer-related research by other agencies of the National Institutes of Health. The American Cancer Society spends about $80 million each year.

How Is the Federal Government Involved in Cancer Prevention and Treatment?

The federal government officially has been involved in the fight against cancer since 1937 when the National Cancer Institute was established to conduct and sponsor research relating to the cause, prevention, diagnosis, and treatment of this disease. A nationwide effort to conquer cancer intensified with the National Cancer Act of 1971. As a result of the National Cancer Program, created by that legislation, more cancer patients are being cured today than ever before, and many others are living longer with improved quality of life.

What Advances Has Research Made During the Past 10 Years in the Fight Against Cancer?

Major advances have been made in recent years in understanding how cancer develops and is spread. Clues to tumor promoters and initiators, which may facilitate the development of cancer, are being found. This knowledge is opening doors to improved methods of diagnosis and treatment of many forms of cancer.

New agents for use in chemotherapy for the treatment of cancer patients are saving and extending lives, and researchers are improving their understanding of the role of viruses in some cancers.

Continued efforts to find new ways to help people stop smoking and to discourage them from beginning the habit are paying off. The National Cancer Institute credits the decline in smoking for the decrease in lung cancer incidence among white males. Knowledge of other possible causes of cancer and the role of such factors as alcohol, diet, and exposure to the sun is increasing.

What Is the Outlook for Cancer in the Future?

Programs to spread knowledge of advances in prevention, diagnosis, and treatment of cancer will play an important part in saving lives in the future. The National Cancer Institute has said that by applying up-to-date knowledge for cancer prevention and treatment, the annual cancer death rate could be cut by as much as 50 percent by the year 2000.

Where Can One Obtain More Information on Cancer?

Cancer Information Service

The Cancer Information Service (CIS), sponsored by the National Cancer Institute, is a nationwide, toll-free number available 8:00 AM to midnight (Eastern time) to answer questions from the general public, patients and their families, and health professionals. Information specialists in CIS offices can provide accurate, up-to-date, and understandable information about cancer causes, prevention, detection, diagnosis, treatment, rehabilitation, and research. In addition, the CIS may know about cancer-related services and resources in local areas. Printed materials on many topics related to cancer are available to callers without charge. The toll-free number of the CIS is 1 (800) 4-CANCER, in Alaska 1 (800) 638-6070, and in Oahu, Hawaii, 524-1234 (neighboring islands can call collect).

Physician's Data Query

Physician's Data Query (PDQ) is an interactive database that provides ready access to information on state-of-the-art and investigational cancer treatments. This online information system is designed to disseminate information on cancer treatment more effectively to the medical community. PDQ is available on the computer system of the NIH National Library of Medicine's MEDLARS system at 2,000 locations across the country. Ultimately, PDQ will be available to physicians through private vendors of computer services, probably via their own regular office computers or word processor equipment. PDQ includes a state-of-the-art statement for each type and stage of cancer, whether standard therapy or investigational. If a standard therapy exists for a specific type of cancer, a range of treatment alternatives will be presented to the database user. Interlinked with the state-of-the-art statements is a directory of oncologists of all disciplines.

National Coalition for Cancer Research
426 C Street, N.E.
Washington, DC 20002

American Cancer Society, Inc.
90 Park Avenue
New York, NY 10016
(212) 736-3030

Glossary

Benign. Not life-threatening
Biopsy. Removal and examination, usually microscopic, of tissue or other material from the living body for purposes of diagnosis
Carcinogen. Any agent that is known to cause cancer in either animals or humans
Carcinoma. Cancer that arises in the epithelial cells that cover external and internal body surfaces

Incidence. New cases of a specific disease occurring during a certain period, usually expressed as new cases per 100,000 per year

Initiator. Any agent that may start the cancer process in animals or humans

Lesion. Any pathologic or traumatic discontinuity of tissue or loss of function of a part.

Lymphoma. Cancer that arises in lymph tissue

Malignant. Tending or threatening to produce death; opposed to benign

Metastasis. Spread of cancer cells from a primary tumor to sites elsewhere in the body

Promotor. An agent that advances the development of cancer once a cell has been damaged by an initiator

Risk factor. An agent or substance that increases an individual's possibility of getting a particular type of cancer

Sources

American Cancer Society
National Cancer Institute

Cerebral Palsy

What Is Cerebral Palsy?

Cerebral (brain) palsy (movement or posture disorder) is a condition caused by damage to the brain, usually occurring before, during, or shortly after birth. The condition is not progressive, it is not communicable, and it cannot be cured.

Cerebral palsy is characterized by an inability to fully control motor function. One or more of the following may be consequences of cerebral palsy, depending on which part of the brain has been damaged and the degree of central nervous system involvement: spasms, involuntary movement, difficulty walking, seizures, abnormal sensation and perception, mental retardation, or impaired vision, hearing, or speech.

The United Cerebral Palsy Association states that cerebral palsy is not a disease and should never be referred to as such.

What Are the Different Types of Cerebral Palsy?

There are three main types of cerebral palsy; sometimes two or all three occur in one person. Spastic cerebral palsy leaves its victims with stiff and difficult movements, athetoid cerebral palsy causes involuntary and uncontrolled movements, and ataxic cerebral palsy affects the sense of balance and depth perception.

What Causes Cerebral Palsy?

Damage to the brain, whether by defective development, injury, or disease, may produce cerebral palsy. Insufficient oxygen reaching the fetal or newborn brain is a ~~~~ cause; this may be due to premature separation of the placenta from the wall of the uterus, an awkward birth position, or interference with the umbilical cord.

Infection of the central nervous system of pregnant women, infants, and young children can also cause cerebral palsy before or after birth. Rubella (German measles) formerly was a frequent cause of cerebral palsy; today that disease is largely under control. Cerebral hemorrhage causes hemiplegia, a spastic form of cerebral palsy, which is the only form that has not diminished in recent years. Acquired cerebral palsy is usually caused by head injury, most often from a motor vehicle accident, a fall, or child abuse.

How Is Cerebral Palsy Managed?

Identification of very young children with developmental disorders gives cerebral palsy youngsters the greatest chance to develop to their fullest capacity. Special attention to movement, learning, speech, hearing, and social and emotional development can help a child with cerebral palsy to live as normally as possible. Sometimes medications, surgery, and braces improve nerve and muscle coordination and either prevent or correct a deformity.

As the child with cerebral palsy grows up, the need for support services may change to include attendant care, continuing physical therapy, special education, vocational training, living accommodations, counseling, transportation, recreation and leisure programs, and employment opportunities.

How Many People Have Cerebral Palsy?

The United Cerebral Palsy Association estimates that between 500,000 and 700,000 Americans have cerebral palsy. Between 5,000 and 7,000 new cases of the disease are diagnosed annually, mostly in newborn infants, and an additional 1,500 preschool-age children acquire the disease each year.

How Much Does Cerebral Palsy Cost the United States?

Cerebral palsy and other disorders of early life cost this country about $3.75 billion in medical care and lost wages in 1986.

How Much Money Is Spent Each Year for Research on Cerebral Palsy?

It is estimated that the National Institute of Neurological and Communicative Disorders and Stroke will spend nearly $46 million on research related to cerebral palsy and other disorders of early life in 1987. The United Cerebral Palsy Association spends about $1 million each year on research.

What Has Research Contributed to the Prevention and Treatment of Cerebral Palsy in the Past 10 Years?

The number of cases of congenital cerebral palsy has declined steadily in recent years, thanks to a combination of prenatal and postnatal care factors. For instance, jaundice of newborn infants is a condition that formerly caused athetoid cerebral palsy in 7,500 newborns each year. Such jaundice is now treated by phototherapy, and the number of infants developing cerebral palsy as a result of the condition is down to about 200.

Lesch-Nyhan syndrome, or hyperuricemia, is a rare and particularly severe genetically determined form of cerebral palsy. A test now enables suspected carriers of the gene to learn whether they are likely to pass this disorder on to their children.

Improved diagnostic tools are making it possible to identify newborn babies and young children who are at high risk of developing neurologic problems, including cerebral palsy, so that the most appropriate treatment can be provided.

Gait analysis clinics enable orthopedists to diagnose leg problems by locating the muscles in which they originate. The use of specially made orthotic devices to correct an abnormal manner of walking has now replaced surgery for many people with cerebral palsy.

What Is the Outlook for Cerebral Palsy?

The United Cerebral Palsy Association predicts that by the year 2000 the incidence of cerebral palsy will be reduced to negligible levels. The association also predicts that improved public education and medical intervention will prevent those cases of cerebral palsy resulting from head injuries caused by accident, child abuse, and neglect.

Improved social acceptance and better support services for the handicapped mean that many people who have cerebral palsy can now live full and productive lives.

Where Can One Obtain More Information on Cerebral Palsy?

United Cerebral Palsy Association
66 East 34th Street
New York, NY 10016
(212) 481–6300
1 (800) 872-1827 (outside New York City)

National Institute of Neurological and Communicative
Disorders and Stroke
9000 Rockville Pike
Building 31, Room 8A06
Bethesda, MD 20892
(301) 496–5924

Glossary

Hemiplegia. A spastic form of cerebral palsy

Lesch-Nyhan syndrome. A severe, genetically determined disorder that is a cause of cerebral palsy

Orthotics. The science that deals with the making and fitting of orthopedic appliances

Palsy. Paralysis; movement or posture disorder

Spasticity. State of increased muscular tone with exaggeration of tendon reflexes

Source

United Cerebral Palsy Association

Coronary Heart Disease
and Heart Attacks

What Is Coronary Heart Disease?

Coronary heart disease is also known as coronary artery disease, coronary atherosclerosis, or ischemic heart disease. These terms refer to a heart ailment caused by a narrowing of the coronary arteries, which decreases the amount of blood flowing to the heart. The narrowing of these arteries can be caused by the formation of plaques of cholesterol and other fatty substances, or it may be caused by a blood clot (coronary thrombus).

What Is a Heart Attack?

A heart attack is an acute manifestation of coronary heart disease. A heart attack is the sudden death of an area of the heart muscle (myocardium), resulting from a reduced blood supply to that area. If the blood supply is cut off drastically or for a long period of time, the injury to the heart can be irreversible; disability or death may result.

When a heart attack is caused by a blood clot, it is called coronary thrombosis, coronary occlusion, or myocardial infarction.

What Is Angina?

Angina pectoris, better known as angina, is the primary symptom of coronary heart disease. It occurs when the heart muscle does not receive a sufficient amount of blood. Angina results in a pain in the chest and often in the left arm and shoulder. It may occur when the blood circulating to the heart is sufficient for normal needs but inadequate for physical exertion or emotional stress.

What Risk Factors Are Associated with Coronary Heart Attacks?

- Cigarette smoking is the biggest risk factor for sudden cardiac death, and smokers have two to four times the risk of heart attack as nonsmokers. When people stop smoking, their risk of heart disease is reduced.

- High blood pressure adds to the heart's workload, causing it to enlarge and become weaker.

- Too much cholesterol in the blood can cause a plaque buildup on the walls of the arteries, which causes them to narrow and eventually close.

- Diabetes can increase the risk of heart attack, emphasizing the importance of controlling other risk factors.

- Obesity, lack of exercise, and stress are considered contributing factors toward the risk of heart attack.

A tendency toward heart disease or atherosclerosis appears to be hereditary. Men have a greater risk of heart attack than women, although women's rates increase after menopause. Black Americans have a greater risk of heart disease because of their higher rate of high blood pressure.

About 55 percent of all heart attack victims are age 65 or older, and 80 percent of those who die are over 65.

How Many People Have Coronary Heart Disease?
How Many of Them Die?

The American Heart Association predicted that in 1987, 1.5 million Americans would have heart attacks and 540,000 of them would die. Heart attack is the leading cause of death in America.

There are nearly 5 million Americans alive today who have coronary heart disease, that is, a history of heart attack, angina pectoris (chest pain), or both.

What Do Coronary Heart Disease and Heart Attacks Cost the Nation?

In 1984, coronary heart disease and heart attacks cost the country $47.1 billion. Americans spent $11.9 billion for medical care for coronary heart disease. An additional $2.7 billion was estimated to be the indirect cost of lost wages due to this condition, and $30.8 billion was the price of lost productivity due to premature death.

How Much Money Is Being Spent on Heart Disease Research?

In 1987, the National Heart, Lung, and Blood Institute allocated $536 million for all forms of heart disease research.

What Research Advances Have Been Made in the Past 10 Years in Preventing and Treating Coronary Heart Disease and Heart Attacks?

A combination of healthier lifestyles and improved medical technology reduced the death rate from coronary heart disease by nearly 25 percent between 1976 and 1985.

How heart disease works

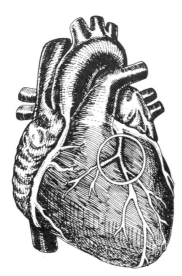

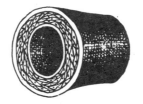

Normal artery

This cross section of a normal artery shows a healthy artery lining which blocks unwanted substances from damaging the artery wall.

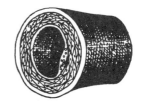

The blocking process begins

The process of atherosclerosis begins with injury to the lining of the artery and the collection of sticky platelets, constituents of blood clots.

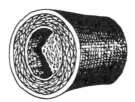

Thickening of the artery wall

Platelets continue to collect and cause the artery wall to thicken, gradually narrowing the opening through which blood can flow.

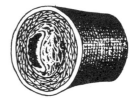

Completion of the process

Platelets continue to accumulate, allowing excess cholesterol and fat to penetrate the artery wall, and resulting in a blocked artery through which little or no blood can flow.

The heart encased in muscle tissue, is fed by several coronary arteries, which are typical sites for the blockages caused by the common heart disease atherosclerosis.

Source: Merrell Dow Pharmaceuticals, Inc., American Heart Association

Source: The Sacramento Bee, September 15–October 3, 1985

Diagnosis. New diagnostic tests have simplified the detection and classification of extent of heart disease. Advances in diagnosis have led to detection of heart disease earlier in its course.

Treatment. A decade ago, the cornerstone of treatment of patients with coronary heart disease was the use of nitroglycerin, which dilates the narrowing coronary arteries, and drugs called beta blockers, which slow heart rate. Coronary artery bypass graft surgery was then available only in university centers for patients for whom medical treatment was not successful.

Today, a wide variety of new drugs is available for the treatment of patients with coronary heart disease, including many different types of beta blockers as well as a new class of drugs called "calcium channel blockers." By judicious use of combinations of these drugs, the number of angina attacks in patients with coronary heart disease can be dramatically reduced. Another major advance has been in the application of thrombolytic drugs (drugs that dissolve clots) in patients with acute myocardial infarction. These drugs may reduce the risk of death and complications in patients with heart attack.

In addition, the technique of coronary artery bypass graft surgery has been considerably refined and can now be accomplished with minimal risk even in severely ill patients. The indications for surgery are more clearly understood.

Prevention. An enormous amount of investigation over the past decade has demonstrated that reduction in elevated blood pressure, reduction in elevated blood cholesterol, and cessation of smoking reduce the risk of death.

Cause and cure. Perhaps the major finding in the past 10 years in coronary heart disease has been the causal relationship between a clot forming in a narrowed coronary artery and heart attack. This finding has opened the question of whether thrombolytic drugs given in the course of heart attack can prevent heart damage or limit the amount of the damage. Recent advances in drugs used to lower elevated blood cholesterol offer the promise of easily followed drug regimens that will dramatically reduce blood cholesterol. It is likely that these drugs will soon be evaluated to determine benefit, risk, and cost.

Where Can One Obtain More Information on Heart Disease?

National Heart, Lung, and Blood Institute
National Institutes of Health
Building 31, Room 4A21
Bethesda, MD 20892
(301) 496-4236

American Heart Association
National Center
7320 Greenville Avenue
Dallas, TX 75231
(214) 750-5300

Glossary

Angina pectoris. An episode of chest pain due to a temporary discrepancy between supply and demand of oxygen to the heart
Aorta. The main trunk artery, which receives blood from the left ventricle of the heart
Arrhythmia. Any variation from the normal rhythm of the heartbeat
Arteriosclerosis. A group of diseases characterized by thickening and loss of elasticity of artery walls
Artery. Vessel that carries blood away from the heart to various parts of the body
Atherosclerosis. A kind of arteriosclerosis in which the inner layer of the artery wall is made thick and irregular by deposits of a fatty substance
Behavior, type A. Characterized by high degrees of competitiveness, aggressiveness, and feelings of the pressure of time; thought by some cardiologists to be a risk factor in development of coronary heart disease
Behavior, type B. More easy going and contemplative, more easily satisfied than type A

Cardiac cycle. The series of mechanical and electrical events associated with one heartbeat; one cycle or beat lasts about 0.9 seconds and includes contraction and pumping, relaxation and filling actions

Cardiologist. A specialist in the diagnosis and treatment of heart disease

Cardiology. Study of the heart and its functions in health and disease

Cardiovascular. Pertaining to the heart and blood vessels

Cerebrovascular. Pertaining to the blood vessels in the brain

Cholesterol. A fatlike substance found in animal tissue

Circulatory. Pertaining to the heart, blood vessels, and the circulation of the blood

Coronary bypass surgery. Surgery to improve the blood supply to the heart muscle when narrowed coronary arteries reduce flow of the oxygen-containing blood, which is vital to the pumping heart

Enlarged heart (cardiomegaly). State in which the heart is larger than normal due to heredity, a large amount of exercise over a period of time, or conditions that cause the heart to work harder, such as high blood pressure, obesity, and defects of the heart or great vessels

Heart attack. The death of a portion of heart muscle, which may result in disability or death of the individual, depending on how much of the heart is damaged

Heart disease. A general term used to mean ailments of the heart or blood vessels

Heart failure. A condition in which the heart is unable to pump the amount of blood required to maintain a normal circulation

High blood pressure. An unstable or persistent elevation of blood pressure above the normal range; uncontrolled, chronic high blood pressure strains the heart, damages arteries, and creates a greater risk of heart attack, stroke, and kidney problems

Infarct. The area of tissue that is damaged or dies as a result of receiving an insufficient blood supply.

Quinidine. A drug sometimes used to treat abnormal rhythms of the heartbeat

Risk factors. Characteristics associated with increased risk of developing coronary heart disease, including high blood pressure, elevated blood levels of cholesterol and other lipids, cigarette smoking, obesity, diabetes, and a family history of heart disease

Vein. Vessel of the vascular system that carries blood from various parts of the body back to the heart

Sources

American Heart Association
National Heart, Lung, and Blood Institute

Cystic Fibrosis

What Is Cystic Fibrosis?

Cystic fibrosis (CF) is an inherited disorder of the exocrine glands, which causes the production and secretion of abnormally thick mucus. The mucus can block passages in several organs, including the pancreas, lungs, liver, and reproductive system. It can interfere with breathing and digestion.

Cystic fibrosis presents a clinically heterogeneous picture, the reasons for which are not known. A majority of cases are diagnosed early in life (birth to 1 or 2 years) with respiratory and gastrointestinal or nutritional problems. In a small percentage of patients, the disease becomes evident only later in life, during early adolescence or adulthood.

What Causes Cystic Fibrosis?

Cystic fibrosis is caused by a defect in a gene, which leads to abnormalities in certain cells and, consequently, the symptoms and effects of the disease. One gets CF from inheriting two defective genes, one from each parent, both of whom are carriers of the *CF* gene. The risk that a child will inherit CF is as follows:

1. If both parents are known carriers, the risk is 1 in 4.

2. If one parent has CF and the other parent has no known family history of CF, the risk is 1 in 40.

3. If one parent is a known carrier and the other parent has no known family history, the risk is 1 in 80.

4. If one parent has a brother or sister with CF and the other parent has no known family history, the risk is 1 in 120.

5. If one parent has a niece or nephew with CF and the other parent has no known history, the risk is 1 in 120 to 1 in 160.

At the present time, there is no way to screen for carriers of the *CF* gene in the general public. However, based on advances made since late 1985, scientists now know that the *CF* gene is located within a particular region on chromosome 7. Using very sophisticated techniques, it is possible in some cases to determine the carrier status of siblings and to perform prenatal diagnosis in certain genetically informative families that already have a child with CF.

With further research advances, it may be possible to screen more individuals at risk of being carriers and, eventually, the general population.

How Many People Have Cystic Fibrosis? How Many Die from It?

There are an estimated 30,000 Americans with CF in 1987. The disease occurs once in every 2,000 births. This relatively small number of CF patients classifies CF as an orphan disease. (See chapter on orphan diseases in this book.)

Cystic fibrosis is the number one genetic killer of children and young adults in the United States.

About 1,000 deaths from the disease occur each year, many of them the result of a lung infection caused by *Pseudomonas*.

The disease affects both sexes equally and is more prevalent in whites (1 in 2,000) than in blacks (1 in 17,000) and is even less common in Orientals (1 in 90,000).

How Is Cystic Fibrosis Treated?

Many medications are useful to CF patients. These include an enzyme to alleviate digestive problems and, for some people, an antacid preparation to make the enzyme more effective. Vitamin and mineral supplements are taken to counteract the difficulty in absorbing these substances. Agents to thin the mucus and bronchodilators to expand the air passages are used by some CF patients. Antibiotics are used to fight the bacteria that frequently infect the lungs of cystic fibrosis patients.

What Is the Cost of Cystic Fibrosis to the Country?

The Cystic Fibrosis Foundation estimates that the cost of medical care for cystic fibrosis patients in 1987 will be $300 million.

There are no reliable estimates on the total cost of the disease, including lost workdays for people with CF who live long enough to enter the workforce, and wages lost to parents who are unemployed, underemployed, or lose time from work to care for CF youngsters.

How Much Money Is Spent for Research on Cystic Fibrosis?

The National Institutes of Health expect to spend over $27 million on cystic fibrosis research in 1987.

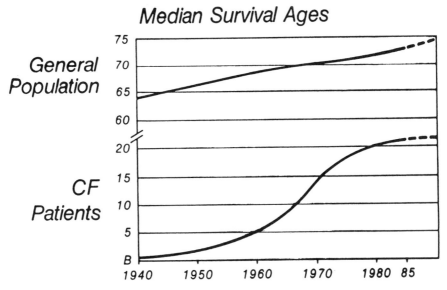

Median Survival Ages

Source: Cystic Fibrosis Foundation

What Advances Have Been Made in Cystic Fibrosis in the Past 10 Years?

Improved antibiotics to control lung infection, particularly that caused by *Pseudomonas aeruginosa*, have helped to extend the lives of CF patients. Enzyme treatments to aid digestion, physical therapy to clear mucus from the lungs, and drugs that thin the mucus all help CF patients.

Genetic research is leading toward isolation of the gene that carries the CF trait and may lead to a test to enable healthy adults to learn whether they are carriers of the disease.

What Is the Outlook for Cystic Fibrosis Patients?

Fifty years ago, infants with CF seldom lived past age 3. Today many reach adulthood and lead very productive lives. Their average lifespan remains, however, very short, about 25 years, although it is increasing.

Where Can One Obtain More Information on Cystic Fibrosis?

National Heart, Lung, and Blood Institute
National Institutes of Health
Office of Prevention, Education and Control
Building 31, Room 4A21
Bethesda, MD 20892
(301) 496-4236

Cystic Fibrosis Foundation
6931 Arlington Road
Bethesda, MD 20814
(301) 951-4422
1 (800) 344-4823

Glossary

Aspirate. The process of mechanical suctioning of liquids or gases from the lungs, often used to remove excess mucus from the lungs of patients with CF

Barrel chest. Enlarged rib cage, caused by some lung diseases, including CF

Bronchial drainage. A form of chest physical therapy used for CF patients several times per day in which the chest is pounded from several different angles and positions to help loosen mucus in the lungs

Bronchitis. An inflammation of the bronchi caused by infection, exposure to cold, or irritants with symptoms of fever and cough

Carrier. A person possessing a single gene for a genetic trait or disorder, such as the *CF* gene

Chromosome. Threadlike material that carries genes, units of heredity; chromosomes are located in the nucleus of every cell; normally, every person has 23 pairs of chromosomes

Chronic. Term applied to any disease or condition of long duration; persistent, not acute (CF is a chronic disease)

Clubbing. Rounded, enlarged tips of the fingers and toes; usually indicates chronic deficiency of oxygen in bloodstream; occurs in CF and congenital heart disease, as well as in some other heart and lung diseases

Dyspnea. Shortness of breath

Exocrine glands. Glands that secrete substances through ducts to surrounding surfaces, including the sweat, salivary, tear, and mucus glands

Hypoxia. Low blood oxygen, may occur in lung diseases such as CF

Malabsorption. Inadequate uptake of nutrients from food between intestines and bloodstream; in CF, due to mucus obstruction of organs in the digestive system, foods are not adequately broken down and absorbed and are not available for use in body maintenance and growth; associated with a common symptom of CF—failure to thrive

Sources

Food and Drug Administration
National Heart, Lung, and Blood Institute
Cystic Fibrosis Foundation

Diabetes Mellitus

What Is Diabetes?

Diabetes is a disease in which the body does not produce or properly use insulin, a hormone needed to convert glucose—a digestive product of sugar, starches, and other food—into energy. It can lead to serious complications that involve many of the body's tissues when high levels of sugar build up in the blood.

What Are the Two Major Types of Diabetes?

There are two major types of diabetes, and they are actually different diseases, according to the National Institute of Diabetes and Digestive and Kidney Diseases. The causes, short-term effects, and treatments for the two diseases differ, but both types can lead to the same long-term health problems. A family history of diabetes increases the likelihood of developing the disease.

Insulin-dependent diabetes, also known as juvenile-onset or type I diabetes, is usually diagnosed during childhood or adolescence. For reasons not yet understood, the pancreas in these patients fails to produce insulin. The person with this disease depends on daily injections of insulin to stay alive. About 500,000 Americans have this type of diabetes.

Noninsulin-dependent, or type II, diabetes is also known as maturity or adult-onset diabetes. It typically develops in people over age 40 who are overweight. In this type of diabetes, the pancreas produces insulin, but the body does not use it effectively. Weight control through proper diet is considered essential to controlling noninsulin-dependent diabetes, and exercise is said to be helpful as well. Oral diabetes drugs and insulin injections are sometimes necessary. Ninety percent of people with diabetes have the noninsulin-dependent form.

What Are Some of the Complications of Diabetes?

When high levels of sugar build up in the blood of a person with diabetes, slow damage can occur to the heart, blood vessels, eyes, kidneys, and nerves. This damage can occur in people who are not even aware that they have the disease.

Blindness. Each year, 5,000 people lose their sight because of diabetes. Diabetic eye disease is the number one cause of new blindness in people between the ages of 20 and 74.

Kidney disease. Ten percent of all people with diabetes develop some kind of kidney disease requiring dialysis or a kidney transplant in order to live. Nearly 25 percent of all new dialysis patients have diabetes.

Amputations. About 45 percent of all nontraumatic leg and foot amputations in the United States are made necessary by complications of diabetes.

Heart disease and stroke. People with diabetes are 2 to 4 times more likely to have heart disease and 2 to 6 times more likely to have a stroke than people who do not have diabetes.

How Many People Have Diabetes?

More than 11 million Americans have diabetes. The American Diabetes Association says that half these people do not know they have the disease.

Each year about 340,000 Americans die from diabetes, and 100,000 more die as a result of its complications.

Who Is Most Affected by Diabetes?

Twenty percent of the people with diabetes are either black or Hispanic. Blacks have noninsulin-dependent (type II) diabetes at a rate 33 percent higher than the general American population, and Hispanics have a rate 300 percent higher. More than 20 percent of the adults in some Native American tribes have diabetes.

There are 190,000 diabetics in nursing homes, about 15 percent of the nursing home population.

What Is the Cost to the Country of Diabetes?

The National Institutes of Health state that the actual cost of diabetes to the country is difficult to estimate because the complications it produces are often listed as the reason for some of the medical expenses incurred.

Thus the $14 billion annual cost to the nation reported by the National Institutes of Health in 1985 is considered a conservative figure. Of that cost, $7.4 billion has been attributed to medical care expenses (though the true figure is thought to be double this amount), and over $6.3 billion is due to indirect costs attributable to disability and premature death among diabetics.

Adult diabetics are hospitalized 2.4 times more often than are adult nondiabetics, and young diabetics are hospitalized at a rate 5.3 times greater than the general population of children. Diabetics average three visits to a physician each year in connection with this disease. Only 10 percent of diabetics report not having seen a physician in over a year.

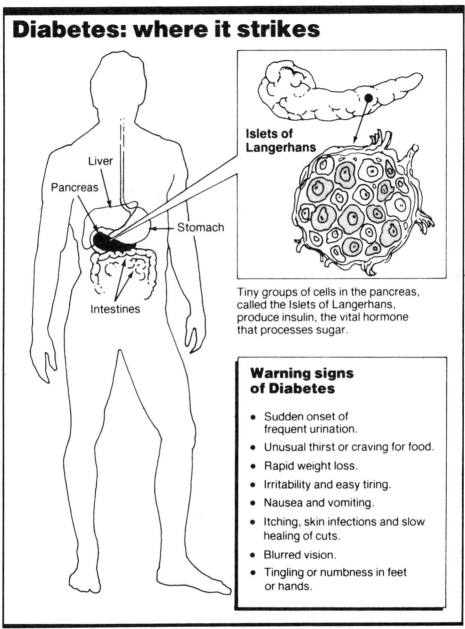

Diabetes: where it strikes

Liver

Pancreas

Stomach

Intestines

Islets of Langerhans

Tiny groups of cells in the pancreas, called the Islets of Langerhans, produce insulin, the vital hormone that processes sugar.

Warning signs of Diabetes

- Sudden onset of frequent urination.
- Unusual thirst or craving for food.
- Rapid weight loss.
- Irritability and easy tiring.
- Nausea and vomiting.
- Itching, skin infections and slow healing of cuts.
- Blurred vision.
- Tingling or numbness in feet or hands.

Source: The Sacramento Bee, September 15–October 3, 1985   Bee graphic/Jim Chaffee

How Much Money Is Spent on Research for Diabetes?

The National Institutes of Health spent approximately $189 million in 1986, and expect to spend $218 million in 1987 on research for diabetes. The American Diabetes Association spent $6 million in 1986, and the Juvenile Diabetes Foundation spent $6.5 million in 1986.

Percent of the U.S. Population with Diagnosed and Undiagnosed Diabetes

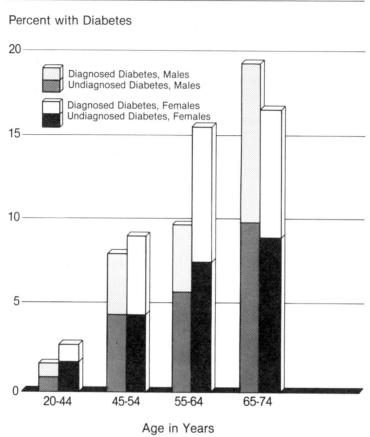

Percent with Diabetes

Diagnosed Diabetes, Males
Undiagnosed Diabetes, Males

Diagnosed Diabetes, Females
Undiagnosed Diabetes, Females

Age in Years

Source: NIH

What Research Advances Have Been Made in Diabetes in the Past 10 Years?

There is no cure for diabetes, but researchers continue to find new ways to control the disease and to prevent or delay the onset of its most serious complications. Among the recent advances are self-blood glucose monitoring, pancreas and islet cell transplants, oral medications, laser therapy to prevent diabetes-caused blindness, and new knowledge about the diet and exercise needs of people with diabetes.

What Is the Outlook for People with Diabetes?

The future for people with diabetes appears promising. Major advances in biomedical research have greatly expanded our understanding of diabetes. Our ability to treat the disease and to prevent or reduce the severity of some of its complications has improved markedly. Nonetheless, current treatment advances, valuable as they are, do not cure the underlying disease, nor do they prevent the most serious complications. Preventing diabetes and reducing the severity of its complications would result in enormous savings in the costs of medical care, hospitalization, rehabilitation services, and economic losses due to shortened lifespan and lost days of work.

Early identification and treatment of people who have diabetes would prevent many Americans from experiencing its serious complications.

Where Can One Obtain More Information on Diabetes?

National Institute of Diabetes and Digestive and Kidney Diseases
Office of Health Research Reports
National Institutes of Health
Building 31, Room 9A04
Bethesda, MD 20892
(301) 496-3583

National Diabetes Information Clearinghouse
Box NDIC
Bethesda, MD 20892
(301) 468-2162

American Diabetes Association
National Service Center
1660 Duke Street
Alexandria, VA 22314
(703) 549-1500
1 (800) 232-3472

Juvenile Diabetes Foundation
432 Park Avenue South
New York, NY 10016
(212) 889-7575

Glossary

Adult-onset diabetes. Noninsulin-dependent or type II diabetes
Aspertame. An artifical sweetener used in place of sugar because it has very few calories

Blood glucose. The main sugar that the body makes from the three elements of food—proteins, fats, and carbohydrates—but mostly from carbohydrates; the major source of energy for living cells, carried to each cell through the bloodstream

Blood sugar. Blood glucose

Coma. A sleeplike state; not conscious; can be due to a high or low level of glucose (sugar) in the blood

Diabetic coma. Severe emergency in which a person is unconscious because the blood glucose is too high and the body has too many ketones (acids); symptoms are a flushed face, dry skin and mouth, rapid and labored breathing, a fruity breath odor, a rapid, weak pulse, and low blood pressure

Diabetic retinopathy. Disease of the small blood vessels of the retina of the eye

Hypoglycemia. Too low a level of glucose (sugar) in the blood; occurs when a person with diabetes has injected too much insulin, eaten too little food, or has exercised without extra food; a person with hypoglycemia may feel nervous, shaky, weak, sweaty, and have a headache, blurred vision, and hunger

Insulin shock. A severe condition that occurs when the level of blood glucose (sugar) drops quickly

Saccharin. A manufactured sweetener used in place of sugar because it has no calories

Secondary diabetes. Diabetes resulting from taking certain drugs or chemicals

Sources

National Institute of Diabetes and Digestive and Kidney Diseases
American Diabetes Association

Disabling Conditions Requiring Rehabilitation

What Is a Disabling Condition?

A disabling condition limits a person's ability to perform one or more major life activities as a direct result of an impairment. The term is usually used to refer to impaired senses or musculoskeletal activity, which may be the result of a brain injury, accident, viral infection, genetic factor, or trauma. Disabling conditions include, but are not limited to, cerebral palsy, vision loss, hearing loss, multiple sclerosis, head or spinal cord injury, stroke, and loss of a limb.

What Is Rehabilitation?

Rehabilitation is the development of a patient's ability to function physically, socially, and psychologically at his or her optimum level.

Where Do People with Disabilities Go for Rehabilitation?

A variety of facilities offer rehabilitation services. In mid-1987, there were 83 hospitals specializing in rehabilitation in the U.S. and rehabilitation units in 524 additional hospitals. Combined, there were about 20,000 hospital beds for rehabilitation care. There were also 115 Medicare-certified comprehensive outpatient rehabilitation facilities (CORFs) and over 500 rehabilitation agencies providing treatment.

Many hospitals provide outpatient rehabilitation services, and many professionals offering rehabilitation services have group and independent practices.

Which Professionals Provide Rehabilitation Services?

A physiatrist is a specialist in rehabilitation medicine and is often the head of rehabilitation departments or facilities. Other physicians, including orthopedists, neurologists, neurosurgeons, urologists, internists, pediatricians, and psychiatrists, may be involved in the rehabilitation of a disabled patient.

Many allied health professionals play an important part in rehabilitation. They include rehabilitation nurses, physical, recreational, and occupational therapists, speech pathologists, vocational counselors, social workers, psychologists, and specialists in orthotic and prosthetic devices.

Some rehabilitation facilities are specialized, providing, for instance, only services for the blind. Others, such as the 176-bed Rehabilitation Institute of Chicago, provide services for people with a variety of conditions, including stroke, head injury, quadriplegia, paraplegia, chronic pain, neuromuscular disabilities, and amputation.

How Many People Have Disabilities?

Various estimates place the number of Americans with disabilities between 20 and 50 million, with 36 million being the most commonly quoted estimate. Because there are many definitions of disability, different sources of data, and inconsistent survey methodologies, it is difficult to calculate an accurate number.

What Does Disability Cost Americans?

It is estimated that our nation's current annual federal expenditure on disability benefits and programs exceeds $60 billion. Federal programs that aid people with disabilities include Social Security, disability prevention programs, transportation, housing, and community-based services for independent living, education, children with disabilities, personal assistance (attendant services), readers and interpreters, and vocational rehabilitation services, as well as matching programs with state and municipal governments.

What Has Research Contributed to Rehabilitation in the Past 10 Years?

Organizations, such as the Rehabilitation Institute of Chicago, are constantly developing new treatment techniques to assist physically impaired people in increasing levels of function and prevention of complications.

Advances in neurology and other branches of medicine have led to the development of new assistive technologies. Present technologies are used increasingly to address the needs of the disabled through new and different applications. As these become more affordable and accessible, they will also have a positive impact on America's disabled populations.

What Is the Outlook for Rehabilitation?

The number of rehabilitation facilities is growing. Reasons for this include the growing population of older Americans who can benefit from rehabilitation services and the number of people whose lives are being saved after experiencing such major health problems as stroke or head injury and now need assistance in becoming independent.

In addition, rehabilitation facilities are exempt from restrictions on Medicare payments, giving hospitals an incentive to move appropriate patients from acute care beds into rehabilitation programs.

One result of the rapid increase in rehabilitation facilities and programs is the shortage of trained medical and allied health care personnel, which the American Hospital Association has predicted will limit the growth of this form of medical care.

Where Can One Obtain More Information on Federal Programs Available to the Disabled?

Clearinghouse of the Handicapped
Department of Education
Room 3132 Switzer Building
Washington, DC 20202-2319
(202) 732-1250

Where Can One Obtain More Information on Organizations Involved with the Disabled?

The President's Committee on Employment of the Handicapped
1111 20th Street, Room 636
Washington, DC 20036
(202) 653-5044

National Head Injury Foundation
333 Turnpike Road
Southboro, MA 01772
(617) 879-7473

National Easter Seal Society
2023 West Ogden Ave.
Chicago, IL 60612
(312) 243-8400

Section for Rehabilitation Hospitals and Programs
American Hospital Association
840 North Lake Shore Drive
Chicago, IL 60611
(312) 280-6132

Paralyzed Veterans of America
801 18th Street, N.W.
Washington, DC 20006
(202) 872-1300

National Spinal Cord Injury Association
600 West Cummings Park
Suite 2000
Woburn, MA 01801
(617) 935-2722

Where Can One Obtain More Information on the Disabled?

Rehabilitation Institute of Chicago
Office of Public Relations and Communications
345 East Superior Street
Chicago, IL 60611
(312) 908-6044

National Rehabilitation Information Center (NARIC)
4407 Eighth Street, N.E.
The Catholic University of America
Washington, DC 20017
(202) 635-5826

Glossary

CORF. Comprehensive outpatient rehabilitation facility
Orthotics. The science that deals with the making and fitting of orthopedic appliances
Paraplegia. Paralysis of both lower limbs and, usually, the trunk
Physiatrist. Physician who is a specialist in rehabilitation medicine
Prosthesis. A manufactured substitute for a diseased or missing part of the body, for
    example, an arm, leg, tooth, eye, or heart valve
Quadriplegia. Paralysis of all four limbs
Rehabilitation. Development of a person's ability to function at optimum level

Sources

American Hospital Association
National Institute of Handicapped Research
National Association of Rehabilitation Facilities

Americans Spend $25.4 Billion on Cigarettes in One Year!
They spend $7.2 billion for medical research
at the National Institutes of Health.

Taking lightly the Surgeon General's warning that "cigarette smoking may be hazardous to your health," Americans spend over $25 billion on cigarettes in one year. At NIH, only $7.2 billion is spent on medical research—only a portion of that money is used for lung cancer research.

Enormous sums are spent on consumer goods in this country.[1]

	(in $ Billions)
Soft drinks	40.2
Beer	35.5
Cigarettes	25.4
Liquor	24.5
Pet supplies	9.3
Chewing gum and candy	9.1
Wine	8.5
Toys and games	6.3
Household paper goods	4.2
Cameras and accessories	3.5
Motor oil	3.1
Photofinishing	3.1
Greeting cards	3.0
Light bulbs	2.4
Household batteries	2.1

Americans spend money on advertising too.[2] Here are some advertising figures of leading companies; these figures represent money spent on the purchase of radio and television time, newspaper and magazine space, and outdoor advertising.

	(in $ Millions)
McDonald's	328
Burger King	167
Budweiser Beer	96
ATT Long Distance Telephone	94
Wendy's Restaurants	82
Kentucky Fried Chicken	81
Miller Lite Beer	76
Pizza Hut Restaurants	72
American Express Credit Card	68
Budweiser Lite Beer	56
TOTAL	$1,124 Billion

[1] *Drug Topics*, July 1985
[2] *Marketing Communications*, June 1987

Leading causes of death by age

Heart disease, cancer, stroke and accidents are the leading causes of death in the United States today. This graph depicts the number of deaths attributed to these causes by single year ages in 1983.

Accidents were the leading cause of death of individuals from age 1 to 36 in 1983. The pattern of 1983 accident fatalities shows a substantial increase in fatalities occurred to persons between ages 13 and 19, rising from 526 for 13 year olds to 2,457 for 19 year olds. Persons aged 19 suffered the greatest number of lives lost to accidents. Accident fatalities gradually decreased from age 19 to age 42, then remained stable from age 42 to age 88.

Heart disease, the leading cause of death overall, was also the leading cause of death of persons aged 59 and over in 1983. Heart disease fatalities peaked at 24,902 for persons 82 years of age.

Cancer, the second leading cause of death overall, was the leading cause of death of persons between ages 37 and 58 in 1983. Cancer deaths peaked at 14,397 for individuals aged 70.

The third leading cause of death in the United States in 1983 was stroke, which overtook accidents as the third leading cause of death of persons aged 55 to 86 and overtook cancer as the second leading cause of death of persons aged 87 and over. Stroke deaths peaked at 6,252 for persons aged 83.

Source: National Safety Council tabulations of National Center for Health Statistics data. ICD codes are 390-398, 402, 404-429 for heart disease; 140-208 for cancer; 430-438 for stroke; E800-E949 for accidents.

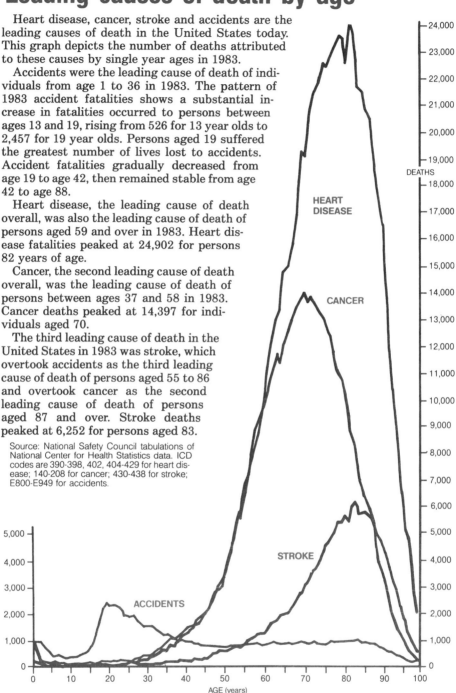

Source: Accident Facts, 1986 Edition. National Safety Council

The stresses of life

The scale of life events

Event	Scale of stress
Death of spouse	100
Divorce	73
Marital separation	65
Jail term	63
Death of close family member	63
Personal injury or illness	53
Marriage	50
Fired at work	47
Marital reconciliation	45
Retirement	45
Change in health of family member	44
Pregnancy	40
Sex difficulties	39
Gain of new family member	39
Business readjustment	39
Change in financial state	38
Death of close friend	37
Change to different line of work	36
Change in number of arguments with spouse	35
Mortgage over $10,000	31
Foreclosure of mortgage or loan	30

Event	Scale of stress
Change in responsibilities at work	29
Son or daughter leaving home	29
Trouble with in-laws	29
Outstanding personal achievement	28
Begin or end of school	26
Change in living conditions	25
Revision of personal habits	24
Trouble with boss	23
Change in work hours or conditions	20
Change in residence	20
Change in schools	20
Change in recreation	19
Change in church activities	19
Change in social activities	18
Mortgage or loan less than $10,000	17
Change in sleeping habits	16
Change in number of family get-togethers	15
Change in eating habits	15
Vacation	13
Christmas	12
Minor violations of the law	11

Source: Drs. Thomas Holmes and Richard Rahe, University of Washington Medical School

Source: The Sacramento Bee, September 15 – October 3, 1985

How people died accidentally in 1985

Type of accident and age of victim

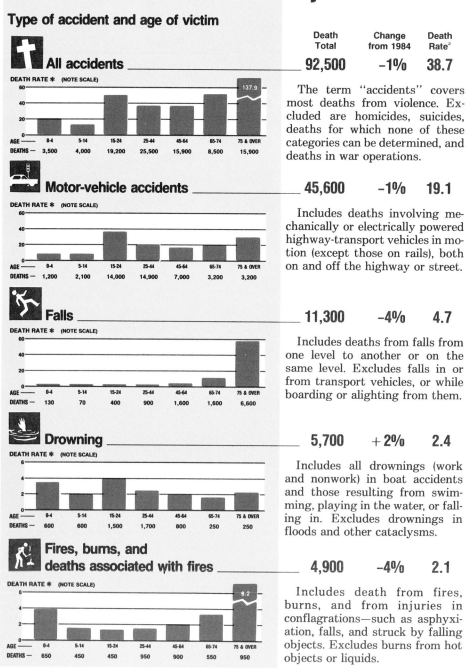

	Death Total	Change from 1984	Death Rate[1]

All accidents _____ **92,500** **–1%** **38.7**

DEATH RATE ✳ (NOTE SCALE)

AGE	0-4	5-14	15-24	25-44	45-64	65-74	75 & OVER
DEATHS	3,500	4,000	19,200	25,500	15,900	8,500	15,900

The term "accidents" covers most deaths from violence. Excluded are homicides, suicides, deaths for which none of these categories can be determined, and deaths in war operations.

Motor-vehicle accidents _____ **45,600** **–1%** **19.1**

DEATH RATE ✳ (NOTE SCALE)

AGE	0-4	5-14	15-24	25-44	45-64	65-74	75 & OVER
DEATHS	1,200	2,100	14,000	14,900	7,000	3,200	3,200

Includes deaths involving mechanically or electrically powered highway-transport vehicles in motion (except those on rails), both on and off the highway or street.

Falls _____ **11,300** **–4%** **4.7**

DEATH RATE ✳ (NOTE SCALE)

AGE	0-4	5-14	15-24	25-44	45-64	65-74	75 & OVER
DEATHS	130	70	400	900	1,600	1,600	6,600

Includes deaths from falls from one level to another or on the same level. Excludes falls in or from transport vehicles, or while boarding or alighting from them.

Drowning _____ **5,700** **+2%** **2.4**

DEATH RATE ✳ (NOTE SCALE)

AGE	0-4	5-14	15-24	25-44	45-64	65-74	75 & OVER
DEATHS	600	600	1,500	1,700	800	250	250

Includes all drownings (work and nonwork) in boat accidents and those resulting from swimming, playing in the water, or falling in. Excludes drownings in floods and other cataclysms.

Fires, burns, and deaths associated with fires _____ **4,900** **–4%** **2.1**

DEATH RATE ✳ (NOTE SCALE)

AGE	0-4	5-14	15-24	25-44	45-64	65-74	75 & OVER
DEATHS	650	450	450	950	900	550	950

Includes death from fires, burns, and from injuries in conflagrations—such as asphyxiation, falls, and struck by falling objects. Excludes burns from hot objects or liquids.

Source: Accident Facts, 1986 Edition. National Safety Council

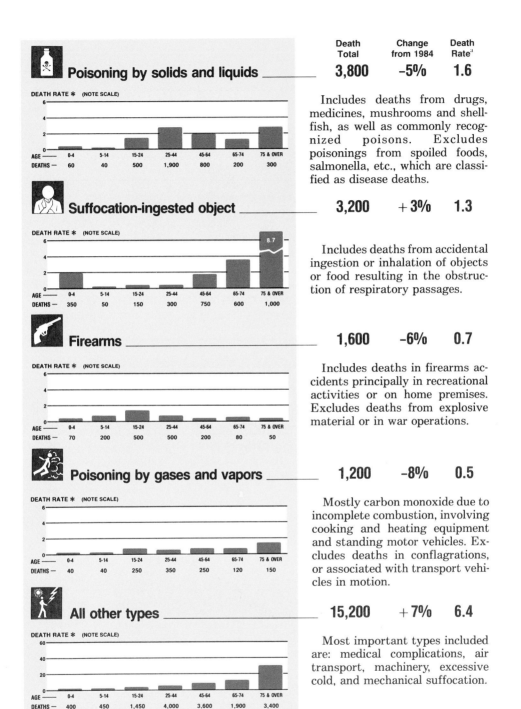

	Death Total	Change from 1984	Death Rate[a]

Poisoning by solids and liquids _____ **3,800** **−5%** **1.6**

DEATH RATE ✳ (NOTE SCALE)

AGE	0-4	5-14	15-24	25-44	45-64	65-74	75 & OVER
DEATHS	60	40	500	1,900	800	200	300

Includes deaths from drugs, medicines, mushrooms and shellfish, as well as commonly recognized poisons. Excludes poisonings from spoiled foods, salmonella, etc., which are classified as disease deaths.

Suffocation-ingested object _____ **3,200** **+3%** **1.3**

DEATH RATE ✳ (NOTE SCALE)

8.7

AGE	0-4	5-14	15-24	25-44	45-64	65-74	75 & OVER
DEATHS	350	50	150	300	750	600	1,000

Includes deaths from accidental ingestion or inhalation of objects or food resulting in the obstruction of respiratory passages.

Firearms _____ **1,600** **−6%** **0.7**

DEATH RATE ✳ (NOTE SCALE)

AGE	0-4	5-14	15-24	25-44	45-64	65-74	75 & OVER
DEATHS	70	200	500	500	200	80	50

Includes deaths in firearms accidents principally in recreational activities or on home premises. Excludes deaths from explosive material or in war operations.

Poisoning by gases and vapors _____ **1,200** **−8%** **0.5**

DEATH RATE ✳ (NOTE SCALE)

AGE	0-4	5-14	15-24	25-44	45-64	65-74	75 & OVER
DEATHS	40	40	250	350	250	120	150

Mostly carbon monoxide due to incomplete combustion, involving cooking and heating equipment and standing motor vehicles. Excludes deaths in conflagrations, or associated with transport vehicles in motion.

All other types _____ **15,200** **+7%** **6.4**

DEATH RATE ✳ (NOTE SCALE)

AGE	0-4	5-14	15-24	25-44	45-64	65-74	75 & OVER
DEATHS	400	450	1,450	4,000	3,600	1,900	3,400

Most important types included are: medical complications, air transport, machinery, excessive cold, and mechanical suffocation.

*Deaths per 100,000 population in each age group.   [a]Deaths per 100,000 population.

Source: Accident Facts, 1986 Edition. National Safety Council

The United States Is Not Keeping Pace With Other Industrialized Nations: A Comparison Of 1980 and 1985 Spending For Non-Defense R&D.

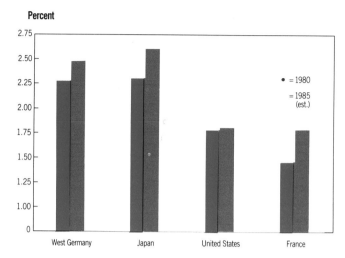

Source: Division of Science Resources Studies, National Science Foundation

Federal Support for Health R&D and Defense R&D (Constant 1975 Dollars) FYs 1975–1986

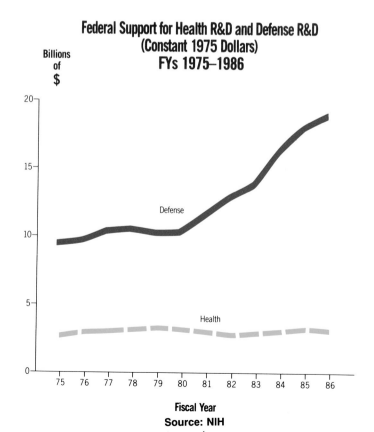

Source: NIH

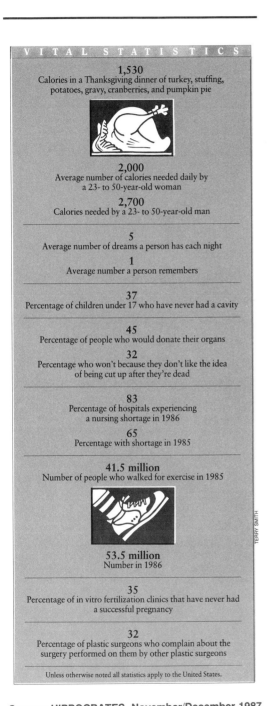

1,530
Calories in a Thanksgiving dinner of turkey, stuffing,
potatoes, gravy, cranberries, and pumpkin pie

2,000
Average number of calories needed daily by
a 23- to 50-year-old woman

2,700
Calories needed by a 23- to 50-year-old man

5
Average number of dreams a person has each night

1
Average number a person remembers

37
Percentage of children under 17 who have never had a cavity

45
Percentage of people who would donate their organs

32
Percentage who won't because they don't like the idea
of being cut up after they're dead

83
Percentage of hospitals experiencing
a nursing shortage in 1986

65
Percentage with shortage in 1985

41.5 million
Number of people who walked for exercise in 1985

53.5 million
Number in 1986

35
Percentage of in vitro fertilization clinics that have never had
a successful pregnancy

32
Percentage of plastic surgeons who complain about the
surgery performed on them by other plastic surgeons

Unless otherwise noted all statistics apply to the United States.

TERRY SMITH

Source: HIPPOCRATES, November/December 1987

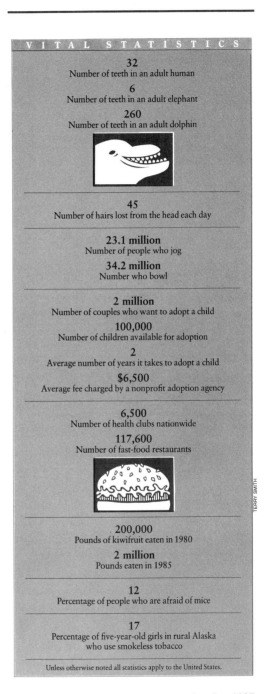

VITAL STATISTICS

32
Number of teeth in an adult human

6
Number of teeth in an adult elephant

260
Number of teeth in an adult dolphin

45
Number of hairs lost from the head each day

23.1 million
Number of people who jog

34.2 million
Number who bowl

2 million
Number of couples who want to adopt a child

100,000
Number of children available for adoption

2
Average number of years it takes to adopt a child

$6,500
Average fee charged by a nonprofit adoption agency

6,500
Number of health clubs nationwide

117,600
Number of fast-food restaurants

200,000
Pounds of kiwifruit eaten in 1980

2 million
Pounds eaten in 1985

12
Percentage of people who are afraid of mice

17
Percentage of five-year-old girls in rural Alaska
who use smokeless tobacco

Unless otherwise noted all statistics apply to the United States.

TERRY SMITH

Source: HIPPOCRATES, September/October 1987

Cancer: The Risks of Where You Live

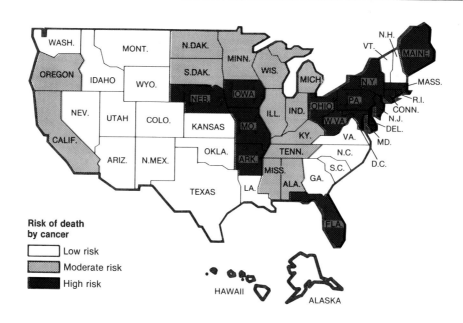

Risk of death by cancer

- Low risk
- Moderate risk
- High risk

HAWAII

ALASKA

NUMBERS INSIDE STATES
IN THOUSANDS

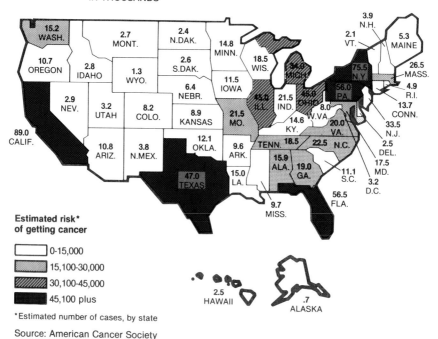

Estimated risk* of getting cancer

- 0-15,000
- 15,100-30,000
- 30,100-45,000
- 45,100 plus

*Estimated number of cases, by state

Source: American Cancer Society

Source: The Sacramento Bee, September 15 – October 3, 1985

Drug Abuse

What Is Drug Abuse?

The National Institute on Drug Abuse defines drug abuse as the use of a legal or illegal drug that causes physical, mental, emotional, or social harm. More specifically, drug abuse can include the use of such illegal drugs as marijuana, cocaine, or heroin, the misuse of pills as recreational drugs that should be used only on prescription, and the overuse of tranquilizers and other prescription drugs by people for whom they have been prescribed.

The spread of AIDS to users of injected drugs via contaminated needles is adding another dimension to the problem of drug abuse.

How Widespread Is Drug Abuse in the United States?

Cocaine. The National Household Interview Survey, conducted in 1985 by the National Institute on Drug Abuse, found that there were 5.8 million cocaine users (people who had used the drug within the past month) in the U.S. in 1985, up from 4.2 million in 1982. This was an increase from 2 percent of Americans age 12 and older in 1982 to 3 percent in 1985. In addition, cocaine users were more likely to report symptoms of dependency on the drug. These data, collected in 1985, do not reflect the full impact of crack, the use of which was not widespread until the end of that year.

Marijuana. The number of people who had used marijuana within a month declined from 11 percent in 1982 to 10 percent in 1985. However, 15 million youth reported using the drug at least once a month, 9 million used it once a week, and 6 million reported using it almost daily.

Hallucinogens. This group of drugs, which became well known during the mid-1960s, includes LSD, PCP, mescaline, and peyote. The already small percentage of the population reporting having used these drugs during the past year continues to decline: among 12 to 17 year olds, 2.6 percent in 1985 compared with 3.6 percent in 1982; among 18 to 25 year olds, 3.7 percent in 1985 compared with 6.9 percent during 1982.

Inhalants. Nine percent of youth ages 12 to 17 reported having experimented with inhalants at some time, and 4 percent reported having used them in the month before the survey.

Heroin. Although current use of this drug was seldom reported in the National Household Survey of Drug Abuse, the Community Epidemiology Work Group of the National Institute on Drug Abuse reports that heroin use continues to be a problem in some areas of the country. The U.S. Drug Enforcement Agency's most recent estimate of heroin use reported that there were 491,000 users and addicts in 1981.

What Does Drug Abuse Cost Americans?

In 1983, drug abuse cost Americans $60 billion. This includes $2 billion for drug abuse-related treatment and medical care, $36 billion on such indirect costs as increased mortality, reduced productivity, and lost employment, and over $21 billion in related costs, such as automobile crashes, crime, incarceration, and social welfare.

In 1986, over 385,000 drug abusers were treated in publicly funded drug abuse programs and facilities, according to the National Association of State Alcohol and Drug Abuse Project Directors.

How Much Money Is Being Spent on Drug Abuse Research?

The federal government, through the National Institute on Drug Abuse, will spend $107 million on research on drug abuse during fiscal 1987.

What Progress Has Been Made in Drug Abuse Research in the Past 10 Years?

While many researchers are investigating the physiologic and psychologic nature of drug dependency, others are working on strategies to educate children and teenagers on the dangers of drug use and developing programs to encourage young people to avoid drugs, along with alcohol and tobacco. The search continues for cost-effective and successful programs to provide help for people who are abusing drugs.

What Is the Outlook for Drug Abuse?

A combination of law enforcement and public education will continue to be necessary to break the cycle of drug abuse, in addition to providing help for people who are already abusing. In addition, it is hoped that measures taken by state legislatures and state medical boards to make it more difficult for physicians to prescribe medications that become drugs of abuse instead of treatment will be effective.

Where Can One Obtain More Information on Drug Abuse?

Epidemiology Branch
National Institute on Drug Abuse
5600 Fishers Lane
Rockville, MD 20857
(301) 443-6637

Glossary

Abuse potential. The property of a substance that, by virtue of its physiologic or psychologic effects, increases the likelihood of an individual's abusing or becoming dependent on that substance

Addict (drug). A person who is physically dependent on one or more psychoactive substances, whose chronic use has produced tolerance, who has lost control over his intake, and who would manifest withdrawal phenomena if discontinuance were to occur

Addiction (drug). A chronic disorder characterized by the compulsive use of a substance resulting in physical, psychologic, or social harm to the user and continued use despite such harm

Chemical dependency. Psychologic or physical dependency on a psychoactive substance

Detoxification. Treatment to restore physiologic functioning after it has been seriously disturbed by the overuse of alcohol, barbiturates, or other addictive drugs

Drug misuse. Any use of a drug that varies from medically accepted usage

Polydrug abuse. Concomitant abuse of two or more psychoactive substances

Prevention. Social, economic, legal, medical, or individual psychologic measures aimed at minimizing the use of potentially addicting substances or lowering the dependence risk in susceptible individuals

Tolerance. Physiologic adaptation to the effect of a drug, which diminishes effects with constant dosages or requires increased dosage to maintain the intensity and duration of effects

Treatment. Application of procedures designed to change patterns of behavior that are maladaptive, destructive, or injurious to the health

Withdrawal syndrome. Signs and symptoms involving altered activity of the central nervous system after the abrupt discontinuation or rapid decrease in dosage of a drug

Sources

American Psychiatric Association
National Institute on Drug Abuse
Alcohol, Drug Abuse, and Mental Health Administration

Emphysema and Chronic Bronchitis

What Are Emphysema and Chronic Bronchitis?

Emphysema is a lung disease characterized by destruction of the walls of the alveoli, or air spaces, in the lung. Its name comes from the Greek word meaning "inflation." This is an accurate description because as the disease progresses, the walls of the air spaces are stretched and destroyed, leaving the person with an enlarged lung and great difficulty in breathing. The small blood vessels in the walls are also destroyed, lessening the opportunities for oxygen to enter the blood, and breathing gradually becomes a more difficult chore.

Bronchitis is an inflammation of the lining of the bronchial tubes. Brief attacks of acute bronchitis, with fever, coughing, and spitting, may accompany a severe cold. Chronic bronchitis is a more serious matter; the condition often develops when acute bronchitis returns each year, lasting slightly longer each time it recurs. Excessive production of mucus in the lower airways leads to the chronic cough that characterizes this disease.

When not properly treated, both diseases can lead to further lung problems and to heart problems.

What Causes These Diseases?

Both chronic bronchitis and emphysema are diseases that seldom strike nonsmokers. The American Lung Association attributes 80 percent of deaths from chronic obstructive pulmonary disease (COPD) to cigarette smoking. Air pollution is often an associated problem. Many people who have one of the diseases also develop the other.

People deficient in the enzyme alpha$_1$-antitrypsin appear more likely to develop more severe emphysema than those with normal levels of this substance in their blood and may get the disease at a younger age. However, even people with this inherited deficiency seldom develop emphysema unless they smoke.

How Many People Have Emphysema and Chronic Bronchitis? How Many Die Each Year?

In 1985, 11.6 million Americans were found to have chronic bronchitits, and 2 million

The lungs: Healthy and diseased

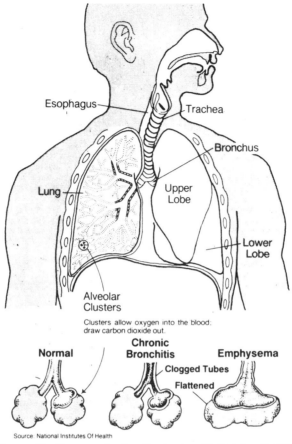

Source: National Institutes Of Health

Source: The Sacramento Bee, September 15–October 3, 1985

had emphysema. Many of these people have both forms of COPD. These diseases caused over 70,000 deaths during 1985.

What Is the Economic Cost to the Country of These Diseases?

Chronic obstructive pulmonary diseases cost this country nearly $10 billion in 1986— nearly $5.5 billion in lost productivity, and over $4 billion in medical care. People with these diseases were treated in hospitals over 406,000 times during 1985.

How Much Money Is Spent on Research on Chronic Bronchitis and Emphysema?

The National Heart, Lung, and Blood Institute allocated $24 million in fiscal year 1987 for research relating to chronic bronchitis and emphysema, and the American

Lung Association spent over $1.7 million in fiscal year 1984–1985 through its awards and grants programs, which are directed toward the prevention and control of all lung .diseases.

What Have Been the Advances in the Past 10 Years in the Prevention and Treatment of Emphysema and Chronic Bronchitis?

Improved methods of educating the public about the health hazards of smoking should have a long-term impact on the number of people who develop these diseases. People who never smoke are unlikely to experience the debilitating effects of these diseases, and those who stop lessen their chances of developing them. Smokers who have chronic bronchitis and emphysema can improve their outlook by stopping smoking. Improved psychologic techniques, along with such aids as nicotine chewing gum, are helping patients and health professionals in this difficult task.

The Bad News: Death Rates for Chronic Obstructive Pulmonary Disease

Age-Adjusted Death Rates
for COPD* Expressed as
Percent Change From 1950 Rate

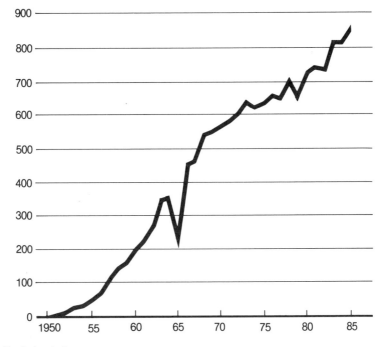

*Includes Asthma.

Source: NIH

The development of rehabilitation techniques, such as respiratory muscle training, can help to make breathing easier for people who have these diseases.

Improved antibiotics help patients to recover more quickly from infections that can complicate these diseases, and immunization against influenza and pneumonia can help to protect these people from further lung disease.

Where Can One Obtain More Information on Chronic Bronchitis and Emphysema and Other Chronic Obstructive Pulmonary Diseases?

National Heart, Lung, and Blood Institute
Office of Prevention, Education and Control
Building 31, Room 4A21
National Institutes of Health
Bethesda, MD 20892
(301) 496-4236

American Lung Association
1740 Broadway
New York, NY 10019-8700
(212) 315-8700

Glossary

Dyspnea. Difficult or labored breathing
FVC. Forced vital capacity; vital capacity performed with a maximally forced expiratory effort
Hypoxemia. A reduced blood oxygen content or tension
Hypersensitivity. A state in which the body reacts in an exaggerated way to a foreign agent, such as an allergen or drug
Hypoventilation. A state in which there is an insufficient amount of air entering and leaving the lung alveoli to bring oxygen to the tissues and eliminate carbon dioxide
RV. Residual volume, the amount of air remaining in the lungs after maximal exhalation; this value is increased in patients with COPD
TLC. Total lung capacity; the sum of all volume compartments or volume of air in the lungs after maximal inspiration

Sources

National Heart, Lung, and Blood Institute
American Lung Association

Hearing Loss

What Is Hearing Loss?

Hearing is the conversion of sound waves in the air into electrical impulses, which are carried by nerves to the brain. The process depends on a series of mechanical and electrical events. When these events are interrupted, the ability to hear either is lost or becomes limited.

What Is Conductive Hearing Loss?

Hearing loss may occur when sound is not conducted efficiently through the outer or middle ear. This is known as conductive hearing loss, which often can be corrected medically or surgically.

Conductive hearing loss may be caused by external blockage, including foreign objects or a buildup of wax in the ears, perforated eardrum resulting from injury or infection, genetic or congenital abnormalities, or otitis media, the middle ear infection that two thirds of preschool youngsters have a least once. Otosclerosis is a hereditary hearing problem caused by an overgrowth of bone in the middle ear. Presbycusis is a hearing impairment of aging, which may be the result of heart disease, high blood pressure, or other circulatory problems.

What Is Sensorineural Hearing Loss?

A second kind of hearing loss is sensorineural, which is caused by inner ear damage or damage in the nerve pathways to the brain. This kind of hearing loss is usually treated by use of a hearing aid. Sometimes hearing loss may be caused by a mixture of conductive and sensorineural problems.

Sensorineural problems include hearing loss at birth. About 4,000 American children are born deaf every year; half of these cases are due to hereditary disorders. Others are caused by prenatal or birth-related problems that cause cerebral palsy, seizures (epilepsy), or mental retardation.

Trauma, including a severe blow to the head, may affect the ear or any of the auditory pathways. Tumors that affect the eighth nerve may affect hearing. Continued exposure to loud noise may affect the hair cells that help to conduct sound. Tinnitus, or ringing in the ears, is a hearing disorder that can torment its victims. Presbycusis is a gradual hearing loss attributed to aging; 25 percent of people over age 65—over 6 million Americans—have noticeable hearing impairment due to this problem, which is a mixed conductive and sensorineural disorder.

How Many People Have Hearing Loss?

The National Institute of Neurological and Communicative Disorders and Stroke estimates that 2 million Americans are deaf and about 15 million are partially deaf.

What Does Hearing Loss Cost Americans?

Hearing loss costs Americans over $23.4 billion each year for medical care and lost income due to disability.

How Much Money Is Spent on Hearing Loss-Related Research?

The National Institutes of Health allocated about $50 million for research related to hearing loss in 1987. This includes funding for investigations conducted by the National Institute of Neurological and Communicative Disorders and Stroke, National Institute of Child Health and Human Development, and National Institute on Aging.

What Gains Has Research on Hearing Loss Made in the Past 10 Years?

Research approaches today are increasingly sophisticated. Numerous neuroscientific tools are being applied in studies of the communicative sciences. These include monoclonal antibodies to identify substances involved in auditory function, intracellular recording from individual neurons in the auditory system, and brain-imaging techniques to provide insight into brain organization and localization of function.

Some scientists are exploring ways to use the body's other sense systems as a means of communication when hearing fails. Vibrotactile aids are under study, and a cochlear implant has been developed that applies electrical stimulation to auditory nerve fibers to improve hearing.

Techniques have also been devised to view the cochlea and vestibule without destroying them. Such advances open the way for studies leading to a more precise understanding of how we hear and what goes wrong when hearing is impaired.

What Is the Outlook for People with Hearing Loss?

The hearing-impaired person today has more learning opportunities and communication aids available than ever before. Legislation enacted in 1973 to prohibit discrimination against the handicapped has meant new horizons for the hearing impaired in employment and education.

Increased awareness of hearing loss, especially through the efforts of voluntary health agencies, has had an impact on treatment and prevention. The public is recognizing that environmental noise can lead to deafness and that hearing loss in the elderly is a disease (presbycusis) rather than a natural consequence of aging. More parents are having their children's hearing tested earlier, allowing quicker intervention and reducing problems of speech and education.

As the elderly population in the United States increases, recognition of presbycusis as a distinct disease should help scientists to focus their research efforts and families to cope with the disorder.

Where Can One Obtain More Information on Hearing Loss?

National Institute of Neurological and Communicative Disorders
   and Stroke (NINCDS)
National Institutes of Health
Building 31, Room 8A16
Bethesda, MD 20892
(301) 496-5751

American Academy of Otolaryngology–Head and Neck Surgery
1101 Vermont Ave., N.W. #302
Washington, DC 20005
(202) 289-4607

National Association of the Deaf
814 Thayer Avenue
Silver Spring, MD 20910
(301) 587-1788

Glossary

Assistive device. Device available from various manufacturers for the hearing impaired to use on telephones, television, doorbells, alarms

Cochlea. The snail-shaped structure of the inner ear that enables sound to be changed into electric current to enter the brain through the auditory nerve

Ménière's disease. A disease that causes loss of balance, dizziness, vomiting, and sometimes hearing loss due to an increase in pressure in the endolymphatic sac (a structure of the inner ear)

Otosclerosis. A softening of the bones of the middle and inner ear that causes hearing
    loss
Presbycusis. A gradual hearing loss attributed to aging

Sources

National Institute of Neurological and Communicative Disorders and Stroke
American Academy of Otolaryngology–Head and Neck Surgery
American Speech-Language-Hearing Association

High Blood Pressure

What Is High Blood Pressure?

Blood pressure is the force of the blood against the walls of the arteries and veins through which it is being pumped by the heart. High blood pressure, also known as hypertension, is the name given to the condition that exists when the heart pumps harder than it should to circulate the blood.

The hypertension threshold recommended by the Joint National Committee on Detection, Evaluation and Treatment of High Blood Pressure in 1984 for an average-sized adult is a reading of 140/90 mm Hg. This is a reduction from the previously accepted rate of 160/95 mm Hg.

Why Is High Blood Pressure a Health Problem?

High blood pressure is a sign that the heart is working harder than it should be and that the arteries are under a greater strain. If the condition is not treated, the heart may continue to work harder and harder, eventually becoming enlarged. When the heart becomes significantly enlarged, it has a hard time working in the way that it should.

In addition, arteries and arterioles may become scarred and less elastic. This is a natural condition of old age, but high blood pressure can accelerate the process. Hardened or narrowed arteries may not be able to deliver the amount of blood the organs need, depriving them of needed oxygen and other nutrients. An additional risk of narrowed arteries is the possibility that a blood clot may become trapped there, depriving part of the body of its normal blood supply. This may result in damage to the heart, brain, or kidneys. The National Kidney Foundation estimates that 18,000 Americans with chronic renal (kidney) disease might have avoided this condition if their blood pressure had been controlled.

What Causes High Blood Pressure?

In about 10 percent of patients, high blood pressure is found to be a symptom of an underlying problem. This is known as secondary hypertension. For instance, a kidney abnormality, tumor of the adrenal gland, or congenital defect of the aorta can all cause high blood pressure. If the underlying problem is corrected, the blood pressure usually returns to normal.

In 90 percent of patients, the reason for high blood pressure is unknown. It is known, however, that being overweight or using a great deal of salt can contribute to the problem. In addition, heredity and age play a role in determining who is likely to develop this problem. The older one gets, the higher the blood pressure is likely to become. Race apparently is another factor in high blood pressure; blacks are more likely to have high blood pressure than whites. This form of high blood pressure is called essential or primary hypertension.

The third and most serious form of high blood pressure, known as malignant hypertension, is extremely severe. A physician can diagnose this problem by looking into a patient's eyes, where the arterioles can be seen. When this condition is discovered, immediate hospitalization usually is necessary. Fortunately, because of wide recognition of the need to control high blood pressure and medicine's ability to do so, this condition is rare in the United States today.

Can High Blood Pressure Be Treated?

Restricting salt intake and keeping weight at normal levels are often effective ways of lowering the blood pressure. But if these methods do not work or if the level of blood pressure is very high, medications are usually prescribed. These may include diuretics to rid the body of excess fluids and salt, vasodilators to widen narrow blood vessels, beta blockers or adrenergic-inhibiting agents to slow the heart rate, or slow channel calcium entry blockers to prevent calcium from constricting the blood vessels.

High blood pressure is seldom cured, so whatever method is used to keep the disease under control—dietary changes or drugs—is usually a lifetime prescription.

How Many Americans Have High Blood Pressure? How Many People Die from This Disease?

Nearly 58 million Americans have high blood pressure or are being treated for it by a physician. More women (33 percent of all women) than men (27 percent of all men) and more blacks (38 percent of blacks) than whites (29 percent of whites) have high blood pressure.

Over 30,000 people died from high blood pressure in 1984, but that is only part of the story. Many additional lives are lost to high blood pressure-caused atherosclerosis, heart attacks, strokes, and kidney failure.

What Does High Blood Pressure Cost Our Country?

In 1984, high blood pressure cost Americans $13.4 billion. Of this amount, $10.2 billion was for medical care, and over $3 billion was for the indirect costs of lost

Blood pressure: what the numbers mean

For individuals aged 18 years or over.

DIASTOLIC BLOOD PRESSURE	CATEGORY
Less than 85	Normal blood pressure
85 to 90	High normal blood pressure
90 to 104	Mild hypertension
115 or higher	Severe hypertension

SYSTOLIC BLOOD PRESSURE	CATEGORY
Less than 140	Normal blood pressure
140 to 159	Borderline isolated
160 or higher	Isolated systolic hypertension

Source: US Department of Health and Human Services

Source: The Sacramento Bee, September 15–October 3, 1985

productivity. In addition, much of the costs of coronary heart disease and stroke can be attributed to high blood pressure.

How Much Money Is Spent Each Year on High Blood Pressure Research?

In 1987, the National Heart, Lung, and Blood Institute allocated over $100 million for research related to high blood pressure.

What Research Advances Have Been Made in the Past 10 Years in the Treatment of High Blood Pressure?

Research has produced a growing number of medications for treatment of high blood pressure, giving physicians and their patients the option to choose the most effective drug with the fewest side effects.

Electronic blood pressure monitors for home use have made self-monitoring possible for those patients for whom it is beneficial.

What Is the Outlook for People with High Blood Pressure?

For people whose blood pressure is under control, the outlook is good. However, the American Heart Association states that the condition is still not controlled in many people. For this reason, educational programs to alert the public to the dangers of high blood pressure are still a high priority for many health experts.

Where Can One Obtain More Information on High Blood Pressure?

High Blood Pressure Information Center
National High Blood Pressure Education Program
Box 120/80 National Institutes of Health
Bethesda, MD 20892
(301) 496-1809

Citizens for the Treatment of High Blood Pressure, Inc.
1101 17th Street, N.W. Suite 608
Washington, DC 20036
(202) 296-4435

Glossary

Aneurysms. Small blisterlike expansions of blood vessels that represent weak spots in an artery and may rupture and cause bleeding or hemorrhage

Arteriosclerosis. Hardening of the arteries; fatty material is deposited in the walls of arteries, which are narrowed

Beta blockers. A group of medications that reduce the force of the heartbeat, decrease the heart rate, and lower blood pressure; also used in treating angina or chest pain resulting from heart disease

Cardiovascular. Refers to the entire system of heart and blood vessels

Coronary. Refers to the heart, e.g., coronary arteries are those arteries that supply blood to the heart muscle

Diuretics. Medications that wash out salt (sodium) from the body and help to reduce elevated levels of blood pressure

Hypertension. High blood pressure

mm Hg. Millimeters of mercury; refers to the height to which the blood pressure pushes a vertical column of mercury

Sphygmomanometer. A device that measures blood pressure

Vascular. Refers to blood vessels

Sources

American Heart Association
Citizens for the Treatment of High Blood Pressure, Inc.
High Blood Pressure Education Program, National Institutes of Health

Influenza and Pneumonia

What Are Influenza and Pneumonia?

Influenza and pneumonia are both infectious diseases of the respiratory system.

Influenza is a contagious respiratory disease caused by a virus. The virus may be spread through the air—when an infected person sneezes, coughs, or even talks—or passed by direct hand contact. The tissues of the respiratory tract become swollen and inflamed, and the patient typically develops fever, chills, weakness, loss of appetite, and aches throughout the body. The patient may feel tired for days after the disease has ended, and the lung tissue may take 2 weeks to heal.

Pneumonia is a lung infection that may have several different causes. The lungs' air sacs fill with pus, mucus, and other liquids, and oxygen cannot reach the blood. Lobar pneumonia affects one lobe (section) of a lung; bronchial pneumonia affects patches throughout both lungs.

What Are the Varieties of Influenza and Pneumonia?

The three classes of influenza-causing viruses are known as types A, B, and C. Influenza A viruses are the most frequent causes of the flu. Viruses in the A and B categories change somewhat every 2 or 3 years, making it difficult for the body's immune system to fight them. Type A makes major changes every 10 to 20 years and can result in a large epidemic, known as a pandemic.

Bacterial pneumonia attacks people whose resistance is lowered, typically infants, the aged, the debilitated, postoperative patients, or those already suffering with viral infections. This is the only form of pneumonia for which a vaccine is available.

Half of all pneumonia cases are thought to be viral. Some forms are not serious, but one type—primary influenza virus pneumonia—is severe and sometimes fatal because the virus invades the lungs quietly, multiplies rapidly, and fills the lungs with fluid.

Mycoplasma pneumonia is usually less serious than other types. It typically affects older children and young adults. Chills, fever, and a sometimes violent cough are its characteristics.

Who Is Most Affected by Influenza and Pneumonia?

Major outbreaks of flu usually occur abruptly. The disease spreads through communities, peaking in about 3 weeks and subsiding after another 3 to 4 weeks. Twenty to 50 percent of susceptible members of the population may be affected, with the highest incidence in children, ages 5 to 14.

The elderly and people with certain health problems are most likely to be seriously ill or to die from the flu or related complications. The following groups are at highest risk for serious illness with the flu and are often advised to receive vaccine:

- Adults and children with long-term heart or lung problems that caused them to see a doctor regularly or be admitted to a hospital for care during the past year

- All residents of nursing homes and residents of other institutions housing patients of any age who have serious long-term health problems

- People of any age who during the past year have seen a doctor regularly or have been admitted to a hospital for treatment of kidney disease, cystic fibrosis, diabetes, anemia, or severe asthma

- Healthy people over 65 years of age

- People who have a type of cancer or immunologic disorder or use medications that lower the body's normal resistance to infection

People who have a particularly high risk of infection and death from this disease are those over 50 years of age and those with chronic illness, such as cardiovascular disease, pulmonary disease (asthma, bronchitis, emphysema), diabetes, cirrhosis of the liver, or sickle cell disease, or people without a spleen or with a nonfunctioning spleen.

Many AIDS patients have developed an otherwise rare form of pneumonia, caused by *Pneumocystis carinii*, as a complication of their disease.

How Many People Get Influenza and Pneumonia Each Year? How Many Die?

During 1985, Americans had 3 million episodes of pneumonia, and close to 65,000 died from it.

There were about 94 million episodes of influenza in the United States in 1985, accounting for nearly 80 million days lost from work and 50 million days lost from school. (This does not mean 94 million people had the flu; many may have had the same disease more than once during the year.) Nearly 2,000 Americans died from influenza during 1985.

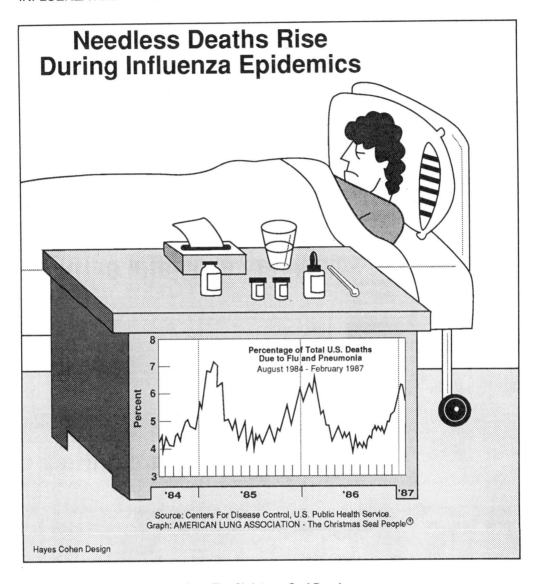

Needless Deaths Rise During Influenza Epidemics

Percentage of Total U.S. Deaths
Due to Flu and Pneumonia
August 1984 - February 1987

Source: Centers For Disease Control, U.S. Public Health Service.
Graph: AMERICAN LUNG ASSOCIATION · The Christmas Seal People®

Hayes Cohen Design

Source: American Lung Association—The Christmas Seal People.

What Do Influenza and Pneumonia Cost the Nation?

In 1986, influenza costs this country nearly $10 billion, most of it ($8.8 billion) in such indirect costs as lost work time.

In the same year, pneumonia cost Americans over $4 billion; nearly $1 billion of this was for direct health care costs, and the rest was such indirect costs as lost time from work (about $1 billion) and loss of productivity due to early death (over $2 billion).

Murderous influenza epidemics

Year	Type of flu	Flu-caused deaths in the U.S.
1918	Influenza A, 2 billion sick, 20 million dead, worldwide	500,000
1957	Asian flu, influenza A	70,000
1968	Hong Kong flu, influenza A, in U.S. 50 million sick	70,000
1975-1976	Victoria flu, influenza A	33,000
1980-1981	Bangkok/Brazil flu, influenza A	50,000

Source: National Institute of Allergies and Infectious Diseases

Source: The Sacramento Bee, September 15–October 3, 1985   Bee graphic/Barbara Stubbs

In 1986, there were 943,000 hospitalizations for pneumonia and 74,000 hospitalizations for influenza.

How Much Money Is Being Spent on Influenza and Pneumonia Research?

The National Institute of Allergy and Infectious Diseases will spend about $9 million in 1987 on influenza-related research and about $23 million on pneumonia investigations.

What Advances Have Been Made in Recent Years in Understanding and Treating Influenza and Pneumonia?

Vaccination against influenza and pneumonia can help some people to avoid some forms of both diseases. As the influenza virus changes, researchers must update the vaccine used to inoculate against the disease.

Antibiotic drugs are used to treat some forms of pneumonia and are sometimes given to people with influenza to prevent pneumonia from developing as a complication of the original disease.

The drug amantadine can sometimes be used to prevent and treat influenza A infections in high-risk people, and additional drugs are being tested for their effectiveness against influenza viruses.

Developments in biotechnology are making possible the identification of specific viruses, which may lead to better methods of treatment.

What Is the Outlook for Patients with Influenza and Pneumonia?

Usually the flu occurs in the United States from about November to April. Although most people are ill for only a few days, some are stricken more severely and may need to be hospitalized.

Patients with pneumonia generally require hospitalization. In untreated pneumonia, the fatality rate is about 30 percent; even with specific therapy, the rate is about 5 percent. The likelihood of death is greatest when infection of the lung is complicated by invasion of the bloodstream by the infecting pneumococcus—a condition known as "bacteremia." In adults, the fatality rate of this systemic condition is approximately 25 percent despite antibiotic therapy. If the infecting organism is the type 3 pneumococcus, the fatality rate rises to 50 percent.

Where Can One Obtain More Information on Influenza and Pneumonia?

National Institute of Allergy and Infectious Diseases
Office of Communications
Building 31, Room 7A32
Bethesda, MD 20892
(301) 496-5717

Centers for Disease Control
1600 Clifton Road
Atlanta, GA 30329
(404) 329-3311

National Foundation for Infectious Diseases
P.O. Box 42022
Washington, DC 20015
(202) 656-0003

Glossary

Amantadine. An antiviral drug used to treat influenza A

Bacteremia. The presence of living bacteria in the circulating blood
Epidemic. A disease attacking many in a community simultaneously
Mutation. A change in the character of a gene that changes the nature of the cell; for
example, the changes occurring over time in influenza types A and B
Pandemic. A widespread epidemic

Source

National Institute of Allergy and Infectious Diseases

Kidney Disease

What Is Kidney Disease?

When working properly, kidneys remove waste products from the body, balance its fluids, release hormones that regulate blood pressure, synthesize the vitamins that control growth, and control the production of red blood cells.

Kidney problems can range from a minor urinary tract infection to progressive kidney failure. Some kidney problems are routinely and successfully treated, but there is no known cure for many kidney diseases, and the result is eventual kidney failure.

Chronic kidney failure, known as end-stage kidney (or renal) disease, is the result of an irreversible scarring process, which causes the kidney to cease functioning. When this occurs, dialysis and transplantation of a new kidney are the only known treatments.

Polycystic kidney disease (PKD) is an inherited kidney disorder, which can also affect other organs. The kidneys become enlarged and have many cysts. About 350,000 Americans have this disease. Adults who develop the disease are usually diagnosed between ages 30 and 50; chronic kidney failure, usually sometime after age 40, is the eventual result. About 10 percent of patients with end-stage renal disease have PKD.

Congenital kidney disease, usually a malformation of the genitourinary tract, may lead to some kind of obstruction, which produces infection or destruction of the kidney tissue. This condition can progress to chronic kidney failure.

Glomerulonephritis (sometimes shortened to nephritis) refers to kidney diseases affecting the filtering part of the kidney. The acute form of the disease usually ends with spontaneous recovery; in its chronic form nephritis usually leads to kidney failure and end-stage renal disease.

Kidney stones are a common treatable disorder. They can result from an inherited condition, a malformation, or a kidney infection or can arise without apparent cause.

Nephrotic syndrome can attack people at any age. When it occurs, there is a large protein loss in the urine. It can be a primary illness or can be secondary to diabetes.

High blood pressure can be a cause or result of kidney disease. Drugs and other toxins can produce kidney damage. Many years of very heavy use of headache compounds can produce this damage, as can some other medications, pesticides and other toxins, and street drugs.

How Many People Have Kidney Disease? How Many Die Each Year?

The National Institute of Diabetes and Digestive and Kidney Diseases estimates that 13 million Americans have kidney and urinary tract diseases each year. Over 93,000 people suffer from chronic renal failure and require either a transplant or an artificial kidney machine (dialysis) to stay alive. It is expected that there will be 106,000 chronic renal patients by 1990.

Half of all men by age 50 and 80 percent of men by age 80 have benign prostatic hypertrophy (prostate problems). Over a million Americans suffer from kidney stones each year. Many people with diabetes eventually develop kidney disease; 50 percent of people with type I (juvenile-onset) diabetes will eventually develop progressive renal disease, leading to permanent kidney failure, as will about 10 percent of those with the type II (adult-onset) form of the disease. Kidney disease is also a potential complication of lupus.

About 80,000 people die of kidney disease each year, approximately 17,000 of them from end-stage renal disease.

What Is the Cost of Kidney Disease to the Nation?

The federal government spends almost $2 billion each year on dialysis, kidney transplantations, and other treatment for 93,000 patients with end-stage renal disease. By 1990, when 106,000 patients are expected to need this expensive treatment, the cost is expected to be nearly $3 billion. Treatment for end-stage renal disease patients is covered by Medicare, without regard to the age of the patient.

The cost to Americans of diagnosing and treating prostate enlargement exceeds $1 billion each year, according to the National Institute of Diabetes and Digestive and Kidney Diseases. This includes the cost of 270,000 prostatectomies.

How Much Money Is Spent on Kidney Disease Research?

In 1987, the National Institutes of Health expect to spend about $111 million for research on kidney disease and related disorders. In addition, the National Kidney Foundation spends about $1.4 million per year investigating the cause, prevention, and treatment of kidney disease.

What Progress Has Been Made in Kidney Disease Research in the Past 10 Years?

Kidney stones can now be treated with extracorporeal shock wave lithotripsy (ESWL) to pulverize the stones with minimal discomfort for the patient. No incision is made, and only a few days of hospitalization and recovery time are required.

Researchers are learning more about the effect of diet on kidney disease. It is now

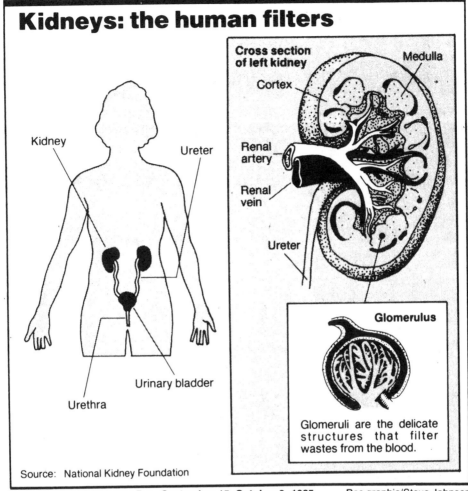

Kidneys: the human filters

Cross section of left kidney
Medulla
Cortex
Kidney
Ureter
Renal artery
Renal vein
Ureter
Urinary bladder
Urethra

Glomerulus

Glomeruli are the delicate structures that filter wastes from the blood.

Source: National Kidney Foundation

Source: The Sacramento Bee, September 15–October 3, 1985   Bee graphic/Steve Johnson

thought possible that a low protein diet might help to slow the progression of kidney failure in some patients, but more investigation is needed before this change in eating habits can be recommended.

Advances in control of diabetes, high blood pressure, and lupus reduce the possiblity that people with these chronic diseases will develop kidney failure.

What Is the Outlook for People with Kidney Disease?

It is estimated the 25,000 Americans could benefit from kidney transplants, but only 7,500 transplants were performed in 1985 because of a shortage of donated organs. Increased public awareness of the benefits of donating one's kidneys at death will increase this number.

Where Can One Obtain Additional Information on Kidney Disease?

National Institute of Diabetes
  and Digestive and Kidney Diseases
Office of Health Research Reports
National Institutes of Health
Building 31, Room 9A04
Bethesda, MD 20892
(301) 496-3583

National Kidney Foundation
2 Park Avenue
New York, NY 10016
(212) 889-2210

American Kidney Fund
6110 Executive Boulevard, Suite 1010
Rockville, MD 20852
(301) 881-3052
National tollfree: 1 (800) 638-8299
Maryland tollfree: 1 (800) 492-8361

Glossary

Acute kidney failure. The kidneys stop working for a fairly short period of time, for a few hours to a few days; usually reversible

Chronic renal failure. Destruction of normal kidney tissue, usually occurring over a fairly long period of time

Dialysis. The process of maintaining the chemical balance of the blood when the kidneys have failed

End-stage renal disease (ESRD). Chronic renal failure, the stage of the disease that requires dialysis or transplantation

Nephrologist. Physician or surgeon who specializes in treating the kidney and kidney disease

Renal. Refers to the kidney

Tissue typing. A laboratory procedure using blood samples to determine if the tissue from a donor's kidney is sufficiently similar to the tissue of a patient's kidneys for a successful transplant

Source

National Kidney Foundation
National Institute of Diabetes and Digestive and Kidney Diseases

Lupus Erythematosus

What Is Lupus Erythematosus?

Lupus is a disease that strikes the immune system, turning it against the very body it is supposed to protect. The cause of the disease is unknown, and its effects can vary. This autoimmune disease causes the body's own cells to attack the lining of joints and other tissues. Lupus is one of over 100 diseases that are considered types of arthritis.

What Are the Major Forms of Lupus?

There are two major classifications of lupus, which may be either variants of the same disease or two separate conditions.

Discoid lupus erythematosus (DLE), or cutaneous lupus, involves only the skin. Patchy, crusty red lesions commonly occur over the bridge of the nose and on the cheeks in an open butterfly pattern. Irregular bald spots may occur on the scalp. This disease is generally relatively mild, but the lesions can be disfiguring. It is thought that the disease can progress to the sometimes more serious systemic lupus erythematosus.

Systemic lupus erythematosus (SLE) is a more generalized disease, with the potential to damage the kidneys, brain, heart, and lungs in addition to the skin lesions of DLE. Periods of improvement and sometimes complete remission may last for weeks or even years between flare-ups. Mortality from SLE was once high, but improved therapy has limited the number of SLE patients in whom serious complications leading to death now occur.

A third lupus disease, subacute cutaneous lupus, is distinguished from DLE by a different pattern of skin lesions and is often accompanied by a mild systemic illness, involving joints and combining fever and a feeling of fatigue.

Who Is Most Likely to Develop Lupus?

Ninety percent of the people who have lupus are women. Blacks, Hispanics, Asians, and some Native Americans appear most susceptible to lupus. Lupus often strikes between ages 20 and 40 but has been diagnosed in children as young as 2 years and in adults as old as 97.

How Many People Have Lupus?

The Lupus Foundation of America says that 500,000 Americans have SLE and another 500,000 may have DLE. Not all experts agree that the disease is this widespread. Lupus has been diagnosed more frequently in recent years, but this is more likely due to better laboratory testing methods and greater physician awareness of the disease than an increased prevalence.

More than 16,000 Americans are newly diagnosed with SLE each year.

How Much Money Is Being Spent on Lupus-Related Research?

The National Institutes of Health expected to spend nearly $10 million on lupus research during 1987.

What Have Researchers Learned About Lupus in the Past 10 Years?

Recent studies of T cell activity and the immune system have brought scientists closer to understanding what happens when lupus occurs. Researchers also are looking for environmental factors that may trigger lupus, possibly in people who have an inherited susceptibility to abnormal immune functions.

The continued development of new nonsteroid anti-inflammatory drugs helps people with SLE because each of these drugs acts somewhat differently. Thus, the more choices available to fight inflammation—one of the major mechanisms of tissue damage in lupus—the better the chance that effective treatments will be found for all lupus patients.

Immunosuppressive drugs, currently regarded as investigational by the Food and Drug Administration for the treatment of lupus, appear to help some patients control the disease.

What Is the Outlook for Patients with Lupus?

Early diagnosis and improved treatment techniques have decreased the number of deaths due to lupus.

Where Can One Obtain More Information on Lupus?

National Institute of Arthritis and Musculoskeletal
    and Skin Diseases
Office of Scientific and Health Communications
Building 31, Room B2B15
Bethesda, MD 20892
(301) 496-8188

National Arthritis and Musculoskeletal and Skin Diseases
  Information Clearinghouse
Box AMS
Bethesda, MD 20892
(301) 468-3235

Lupus Foundation of America
1717 Massachusetts Ave., N.W.
Washington, DC 20036
(202) 328-4550

Glossary

Antibody. Serum protein made in response to an antigen

Antigen. Protein that stimulates formation of antibodies

Autoantibody. Antibody directed against the body's own tissue

Autoimmune. Sensitive to oneself; a person's body makes antibodies against some of
  its own cells

Butterfly rash. A double-wing-shaped skin rash around the nose and cheeks, highly
  suggestive of lupus

Collagen disease. Diseases characterized by inflammation of connective tissues, especially the skin and joints—rheumatoid arthritis, SLE, scleroderma, Sjögren's
  syndrome, juvenile rheumatoid arthritis, also usually synonymous with rheumatic
  disease

Complement protein. Regulator molecule of the immune response

Connective tissue. Substance that binds the body together, like a body glue, the most
  widespread and abundant tissue in the body

Cutaneous lesions. Visible changes in skin that are abnormal; rashes, sores, or scars

Discoid lupus erythematosus (DLE). Cutaneous lupus, affecting only the skin

Exacerbation. Recurrence of symptoms

Flare. Exacerbation

Immune complexes. Specific combination of antibodies with their corresponding antigens

Immune mediated. Produced by the immune system, i.e., antibodies and lymphocytes

Immune response. Response of the body's immune system to antigens

Immunity. Power to resist infection

Mixed connective tissue disease. Consisting of two or more of the connective tissue
  diseases, e.g., lupus, polymyositis, scleroderma

Renal. Pertaining to the kidneys

Sjögren's syndrome. Autoimmune disease characterized by dryness of the mouth and
  eyes

Spontaneous remission. Marked improvement in a disease that occurs without medical intervention

Systemic lupus erythematosus (SLE). Generalized lupus, affecting kidneys, brain, heart, lungs, and skin

T cells. White blood cells processed in the thymus and responsible for cell-mediated immunity

Sources

National Institute of Arthritis and Musculoskeletal and Skin Diseases
Lupus Foundation of America

Mental Illness

What Is Mental Illness?

A mental illness is an impairment in functioning due to a social, psychologic, genetic, physical, chemical, or biologic disturbance. Just as other diseases have specific symptoms and treatments, mental illnesses usually can be accurately diagnosed and effectively treated.

Many people seek the services of mental health professionals—psychiatrists, psychologists, social workers, marriage and family counselors—for what have been called problems in living. They want help in improving marital relationships, relating to peers, coping on the job, boosting self-confidence, or dealing with stress. More serious in terms of the intensity of treatment needed are the following mental illnesses:

Anxiety disorders, including phobias, panic disorders, and obsessive-compulsive disorders. An estimated 13 million Americans, or 8 percent of the population, have these kinds of disorders, according to a 1980–1982 study. Phobias are said to be America's most common mental disorder; over 5 percent of the population have some form of this condition.

Depression. About 5 percent of Americans are thought to have this disorder, known technically as affective disorder. Depression is a mental disorder with a lasting altered mood, for no obvious external cause. Treatment may be by antidepressant medication or psychotherapy or a combination of the two. Treatment is important because people with depression may become suicidal.

Abuse or dependence on alcohol or drugs. At least 6 percent of the population is said to have this problem; in about 80 percent of the cases, alcohol is the problem.

Schizophrenia. About 1 percent of the American population has schizophrenia, a disease characterized by delusions, hallucinations, or thought disturbances. The degree of impairment from this disorder varies. Some patients may need institutional care, whereas others may function well, often with the help of regular medication.

Antisocial personality disorders. About 1 percent of the population is said to have this problem, one of a group of mental problems known as personality disorders. Antisocial personality disorder may be characterized by superficial charm, refusal to accept guilt, substance abuse, and inability to function as a responsible parent.

What Is the Relationship Between Mental and Physical Illness?

Many health professionals are giving increased attention to the interrelationship between mental and physical illnesses. For instance, psychologists often treat sleep disorders and chronic pain, and many experts believe that both these conditions are sometimes related to the mental illness of depression. There is a growing recognition of the importance of stress control for patients with high blood pressure and heart disease.

How Are Mental and Emotional Illness Treated?

A variety of professionals, including primary care physicians, psychiatrists, psychologists, social workers, nurses, marriage and family counselors, and other specialists with various levels of training, treat patients with mental and emotional illness.

Today, the vast majority of mental health care is given on an outpatient basis. Of 5.6 million episodes of care, 18 percent were for inpatients or residential treatment, 77 percent were for outpatient care, and 5 percent were for partial care. In 1955, 77 percent of the care was inpatient.

How Many Americans Have Mental Illnesses?

During any 6-month period, nearly 30 million adult Americans (over 18 percent of the population) suffer from one or more mental illnesses. But less than 20 percent of people with a mental illness receive any kind of treatment for it during a 6-month period, from either a mental health specialist or general medical physicians.

A 1983 survey of 250,000 primary care physicians, psychiatrists, psychologists, and social workers found that patients with the following mental and emotional illnesses had been seen during one 60-day period (note that these are patients seen for the condition; far more people have the condition):

Schizophrenia, mania, and major depression	2 million
Substance abuse and alcoholism	1.5 million
Somatoform and psychosexual disorders	1.1 million
Neurosis, anxiety, and personality disorders	3.3 million
Relationship problems	2 million
Other conditions	1.5 million

What Is the Cost to Our Nation of Mental Illness?

In 1983, the total cost of mental illness to the nation was estimated to be nearly $73 billion. This included $33.4 billion for direct costs of diagnosis, treatment, and support services, $37.1 billion for such indirect costs as reduced productivity, lost employment, and increased mortality, and $2.2 billion in such related costs as automobile accidents, crime, incarceration, and social welfare.

In 1983, $80 billion was spent for treatment of mental illness, including treatment for drug and alcohol abuse. This was 14.2 percent of the nation's total medical expenditure for that year.

How Much Money Is Being Spent on Research Relating to Mental and Emotional Illness?

The National Institute of Mental Health will spend about $247 million on research in 1987.

What Have Researchers Learned About Mental and Emotional Illness in the Past 10 Years?

Progress continues to be made in understanding the physiologic and biochemical bases of mental illness, sometimes narrowing the gap between which diseases are physical and which are mental. In addition, the physiologic effects of such mental states as stress are being more widely recognized.

At the same time that new medications have been developed and brought to market, researchers continue to learn how these drugs can be used most effectively, in many cases combining drugs with psychotherapy.

What Is the Outlook for People with Mental and Emotional Illness?

Despite wide popular interest in psychology and mental health, reflected by articles on related subjects in popular magazines and the growing number of radio and television programs featuring psychologists and other mental health professionals, many people with mental illness remain undiagnosed and untreated.

The growth of employee assistance programs, which often refer workers to professionals for assistance with mental illness, may help some people to get the care they should have. Some experts believe that better insurance coverage for treatment of mental illness would enable many more people to obtain the help they need.

Increased research is taking place to determine the chemical and hormonal causes of depression and anxiety. New therapeutic modalities, including the use of psychopharmaceuticals, have shown benefit and promise.

Where Can One Obtain More Information on Mental Illness?

American Psychiatric Association
1400 K Street, N.W.
Washington, DC 20005
(202) 682-6000

National Institute of Mental Health
Office of Scientific Information
15-105 Parklawn Building, Room 15105
5600 Fishers Lane
Rockville, MD 20857
(301) 443-3600

Glossary

Anxiety. Apprehension, tension, or uneasiness from anticipated danger, the source of
    which is largely unknown or unrecognized
Autism. Developmental disability caused by a physical disorder of the brain appearing
    during the first 3 years of life; symptoms include disturbances in physical, social,
    and language skills, abnormal responses to sensations, and abnormal ways of
    relating to people, objects, and events
Behavior therapy. Mode of treatment that focuses on modifying observable and quan-
    tifiable behavior by means of systematic manipulation of the environmental and
    behavioral variables thought to be functionally related to the behavior
Delusion. A false belief firmly held despite evidence to the contrary
Depression. When used to describe a mood, which may be a normal state, depression
    refers to feelings of sadness, despair, and discouragement. Depression may be a
    symptom in a variety of mental or physical disorders, a syndrome of associated
    symptoms secondary to an underlying disorder, or a specific mental disorder
Hallucination. A sensory perception in the absence of an actual external stimulus
Mania. An inordinately intense enthusiasm, craze
Manic-depressive illness. Also known as bipolar disorder, in which there are episodes
    of both mania and depression
Personality disorders. Deeply ingrained, inflexible, maladaptive patterns of relating,
    perceiving, and thinking of sufficient severity to cause either impaired functioning
    or distress
Psychotherapy. A process by which a person who wishes to relieve symptoms or
    resolve problems in living or is seeking personal growth enters into an implicit
    or explicit contract to interact in a prescribed way with a psychotherapist

Schizophrenia. A large group of disorders manifested by characteristic disturbances of language and communication, thought perception, affect, and behavior that last longer than 6 months

Sources

American Psychiatric Association
American Psychological Association
National Institute of Mental Health

Multiple Sclerosis

What Is Multiple Sclerosis?

Multiple sclerosis (MS) is a chronic neurologic disease caused by the breaking down of the myelin, the fatty sheath that insulates the nerve fibers of the brain and spinal cord. As the protective myelin disintegrates, the nerve signals become distorted or fail completely. Symptoms vary, depending on what portion of the brain or spinal cord is affected; they may include weakness, loss of coordination, double vision, slurred speech, or uncontrollable tremors. Loss of bladder control, decline in sexuality, and paralysis may also occur.

Multiple sclerosis is not contagious. It is not a mental disease, although some patients have trouble with memory and decision making. It is seldom fatal. Recent research has shown that MS is probably an autoimmune disease, possibly triggered by a childhood infection.

What Course Does the Disease Follow?

Multiple sclerosis affects each patient differently, but four patterns to the disease have been identified. In its benign form, there is no permanent functional disability (20 percent of patients); a pattern of exacerbations (attacks) followed by remissions occurs in 20 percent of people with MS; exacerbating/remitting disease with gradually progressive disability occurs in 40 percent of people with MS; and steadily worsening (known as chronic progressive) disease from the outset is the pattern for 10 to 20 percent of MS patients.

Who Gets Multiple Sclerosis?

Multiple sclerosis has been known to strike as early as age 10 or as late as age 60, but most often the disease is diagnosed in people between ages 20 and 40. Women get the disease earlier than men and twice as often. Siblings of MS patients appear more prone to getting the disease.

Multiple sclerosis occurs most often in the northern United States, Canada, England, northern Europe, southern Australia, and New Zealand.

Common Symptoms of Multiple Sclerosis

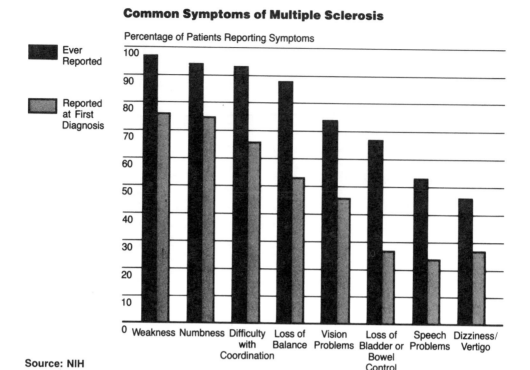

Percentage of Patients Reporting Symptoms

Ever Reported

Reported at First Diagnosis

Weakness Numbness Difficulty with Coordination Loss of Balance Vision Problems Loss of Bladder or Bowel Control Speech Problems Dizziness/ Vertigo

Source: NIH

How Many Americans Have Multiple Sclerosis?

The National Multiple Sclerosis Society estimates that about 250,000 Americans have this disease.

How Much Does Multiple Sclerosis Cost This Country?

The National Multiple Sclerosis Society says Americans spent over $402 million on medical care for MS in 1985; in the same year, nearly $1.4 billion in lost earnings was attributed to MS.

Part of the reason for the high cost of MS is that most of its victims live a near-normal lifespan. Because the disease strikes while its victims are young, they may be prevented from reaching their full earning power and sometimes have high medical expenses for many years.

How Much Money Is Spent on Multiple Sclerosis Research?

The National Institutes of Health budgeted about $76 million for research on MS and related disorders in 1987. Investigations are carried out in the National Institute of

Neurological and Communicative Disorders and Stroke, the National Institute of Allergy and Infectious Diseases, and the Division of Research Resources.

In addition, the National Multiple Sclerosis Society will spend nearly $7 million on research in 1987.

What Advances Have Been Made in Multiple Sclerosis Research in the Past 10 Years?

Researchers are pursuing many avenues that may lead to a better understanding of why MS strikes its victims and perhaps indicate a way to prevent the disease. They are also seeking an accurate, inexpensive way to diagnose the disease when it is suspected.

Because there is no cure for MS, physicians often prescribe drugs that have been found to shorten an attack or lessen some of its symptoms. Some patients find relief from spasticity through muscle relaxants and tranquilizers, some are helped by alleviation of pain through strong prescription pain killers, and some find the drug amantadine effective in fighting fatigue. Other drugs are undergoing clinical trials in the hope that they will offer relief from MS symptoms.

What Is the Outlook for People with Multiple Sclerosis?

Prospects for leading a productive life are improving for MS patients because of better therapeutic treatment and greater ability of physicians to manage the disease and alleviate symptoms.

Where Can One Obtain More Information on Multiple Sclerosis?

National Institute of Neurological and Communicative Disorders and Stroke
Public Liaison Section
Building 31, Room 8A06
National Institutes of Health
Bethesda, MD 20894
(301) 496-5924

National Multiple Sclerosis Society
205 East 42nd Street
New York, NY 10017
1 (800) 637-6303
(212) 986-3240

Glossary

ACTH. Adrenocorticotropic hormone, a natural product of the body, used as a short-term anti-inflammatory agent; used to alleviate exacerbations for many MS patients

Autoimmune response. Abnormal reaction of the body's immune system, directed against its own tissues, organs, or cells

Demyelination. Loss of myelin, the fatty sheath that insulates nerve fibers, resulting in blocked or altered transmission

Diplopia. Double vision

Exacerbation. A temporary period of increased MS symptoms, lasting days, weeks, or months

MRI (or NMR). Magnetic resonance imaging or nuclear magnetic resonance, a complex method of producing a map of internal tissues, such as the brain

Myelin sheath. Fatty insulation covering the nerve fibers throughout the nervous system

Nystagmus. Involuntary, rapid movements of the eyeball horizontally, vertically, or rotationally

Paresthesias. Pins-and-needles or tingling sensations in any part of the body

Plaques. Patchy areas of inflammation and demyelination, which in time become sclerosed (scarred)

Remission. A period when symptoms of a disease diminish or disappear entirely

Sclerosis. Scarring

Spasticity. A stiffness or muscle tightness, usually in legs

Source

National Multiple Sclerosis Society

Orphan Diseases

What Is an Orphan Disease?

An orphan disease is an illness that affects fewer than 200,000 Americans. The National Organization for Rare Disorders says that there are over 5,000 such diseases, over half of them genetic diseases.

Some orphan diseases are well known and are, in fact, described in chapters of this book (including AIDS, cystic fibrosis, sickle cell disease, and sudden infant death syndrome). Others are less frequently occurring, specific forms of diseases that fall within some of the broader chapters of this book (including cancer, arthritis, and mental illness). Cerebral palsy, lupus erythematosus, and multiple sclerosis (see chapters in this book) are considered orphan diseases by the National Organization for Rare Disorders despite the larger numbers of people who have these conditions.

Examples of better-known orphan diseases include amytrophic lateral sclerosis (Lou Gehrig's disease), narcolepsy, cystinosis, Huntington's disease, Gaucher's disease, retinitis pigmentosa, and Legionnaire's disease.

How Many Americans Have Orphan Diseases?

More than 5 million Americans have one of these rare, debilitating conditions.

Why the Name "Orphan?"

The Orphan Drug Act was passed on January 4, 1983, with the objective of making drug treatments for rare disorders more available to the people in need of them. During the 1970s, new treatments for some rare disorders were discovered by academic scientists, but they remained undeveloped until passage of the Orphan Drug Act.

These drugs had been perceived by the pharmaceutical industry as being unprofitable because the cost of development would far outweigh the potential for profit. While drugs for more common health conditions were being developed and sold to millions of people at a great profit, drugs for rare diseases remained orphans waiting for adoption so that they could be developed, manufactured, and marketed and thus become available to the people who needed them.

How Does the Orphan Drug Act Help?

This Act provides incentives to pharmaceutical companies to develop orphan drugs. These incentives include a special designation for experimental drugs used to treat diseases affecting less then 200,000 Americans. When a drug is designated an "orphan," the FDA provides protocol preparation assistance, tax credits for the cost of clinical research, a faster approval process, and 7 years of exclusive marketing rights for the drug's manufacturer.

In October 1984, the Orphan Drug Act was amended to include diseases or conditions that affect more than 200,000 people but for which there is no reasonable expectation that a drug will be developed and made available in the U.S. because of economic considerations.

Has the Orphan Drug Act Accomplished Its Purpose?

By mid-1987, 130 drugs had been granted orphan status by the FDA, and 40 of them had been approved for marketing. Among the drugs designated as orphans are AZT (trade name Retrovir) for use in treating certain cases of AIDS, Naltrexone for treatment of narcotic addiction, and cyclosporine, an immunosuppressant used to prevent organ transplant rejection.

How Much Money Is Spent on Orphan Drug Research?

The Orphan Drug Act authorized $4 million per year to support scientific research grants on new therapies for rare disorders. In 1986, the Food and Drug Administration awarded 21 orphan product research grants totalling $2.8 million. The NIH also provides varying degrees of support for most orphan diseases depending on quality of research and available opportunities.

What Is the Outlook for Orphan Diseases?

The U.S. Department of Health and Human Services has created a National Commission on Orphan Diseases, which will report to Congress on the prospects for improved treatment for these diseases.

Where Can One Obtain More Information on Orphan Diseases?

Pharmaceutical Manufacturers Association
Commission on Drugs for Rare Diseases
1100 15th Street, N.W. Suite 900
Washington, DC 20005
(202) 835-3561

National Organization for Rare Disorders, Inc.
P.O. Box 8923
New Fairfield, CT 06812
(203) 746-6518

Office of Orphan Development Products
Federal Drug Administration
Room 12A-40 Mail Code HF 35
5600 Fishers Lane
Rockville, MD 20857
(301) 443-4903

Glossary

Amyotrophic lateral sclerosis (Lou Gehrig's disease). A disease causing muscular
   atrophy, twitching, and spastic irritability of muscles
Cystinosis. Cystine storage disease
Gaucher's disease. Familial splenic anemia, occurring most severely in infants
Huntington's disease. A chronic, progressive disorder characterized by spasmodic
   involuntary movements in the face and extremities, followed by gradual loss of
   mental faculties
Legionnaire's disease. An acute, infectious disease with influenza-like symptoms
Narcolepsy. A sudden, uncontrollable disposition to sleep
Orphan drug. A drug used in treatment of rare disorders (orphan diseases)
Retinitis pigmentosa. Noninflammatory degenerative disease of the retina with pig-
   mentary infiltration

Sources

Pharmaceutical Manufacturers Association Commission on Drugs
for Rare Diseases
National Organization for Rare Disorders, Inc.
Food and Drug Administration

Sickle Cell Anemia

What Is Sickle Cell Anemia?

Sickle cell anemia is an inherited disorder of the red blood cells. A person who has sickle cell disease, as the condition is sometimes called, has red blood cells that become sickle shaped instead of round when they have given their oxygen up to the body.

Why Is Sickle Cell Anemia a Serious Disease?

These misshapen blood cells do not flow through the small blood vessels easily and may clog them, reducing the nourishment that flows to the part of the body the vessel serves. This blockage can result in painful crises or lead to such other serious complications as kidney disease and stroke, heart, lung, and bone damage, and leg ulcers. Infections are also more frequent and more dangerous in people with sickle cell disease.

Sickle cells are more fragile than normal blood cells and tend to be destroyed more rapidly. Thus the person becomes anemic because there are too few red blood cells.

What Is Sickle Cell Trait?

People with sickle cell trait carry the recessive gene that can cause sickle cell anemia. The disease will occur in an offspring only if one carrier mates with another carrier of the trait. Because the gene is recessive, not all of the children of people with sickle cell trait will inherit the disease. People who carry the trait do not have the disease.

Who Gets Sickle Cell Anemia?

Like many hereditary diseases, certain ethnic groups are most likely to be carriers of sickle cell trait. In the U.S., it is largely blacks who have the potential to pass on the disease. About 1 of 10 black Americans has sickle cell trait.

How Many Americans Have Sickle Cell Anemia?

About 50,000 people in the U.S. are thought to have sickle cell anemia. Because sickle cell disease can mimic many other disorders, many people who have the disease may not know it until they are adults or may never have the underlying cause of their recurrent illnesses diagnosed.

What Does Sickle Cell Anemia Cost the Country?

Many people with sickle cell anemia have more frequent health problems than the rest of the population, but because the expenditure is rarely for treatment of sickle cell disease itself, there is no real information on the cost of the disease.

Payment for medical care of people who have been diagnosed as having sickle cell disease is frequently a problem, because many health insurers consider it a preexisting medical condition.

How Much Money Is Spent on Sickle Cell Anemia Research?

The National Heart, Lung, and Blood Institute budgeted $30 million for sickle cell research in 1987.

What Have Researchers Learned About Sickle Cell Anemia in the Past 10 Years?

A major potential advance in the care of children with sickle cell disease is strong evidence supporting the use of daily doses of oral penicillin to prevent the bacterial infections that can be life-threatening.

The recognition that this treatment can significantly reduce episodes of serious infectious illness in young children has convinced many experts that routine screening for sickle cell anemia should be performed at birth so that infants with the disease can be treated.

What Is the Outlook for Sickle Cell Anemia?

Recognition of the needs of sickle cell anemia patients, along with better medical treatment, has lengthened the lifespan for many people with the disease. Many people with sickle cell anemia now live into their 60s, according to the Center for Sickle Cell Disease at Howard University.

Screening infants at birth so that those who have the disease can be treated appropriately can decrease both the episodes of acute illness and the number of early deaths from conditions related to the disease.

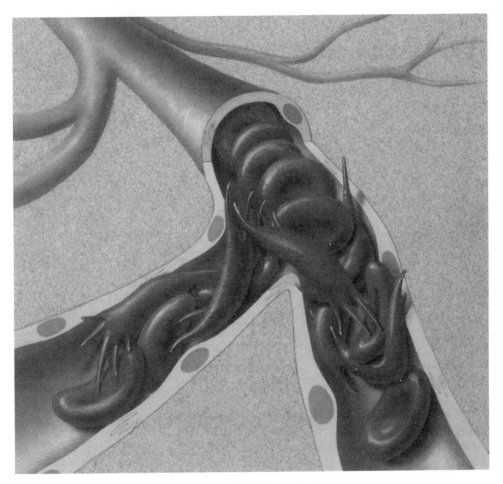

Abnormal sickled red cells block the flow of blood in a capillary.
Source: National, Heart, Lung, and Blood Institute

Like most genetic disorders, sickle cell disease cannot be cured. However, genetic counseling for couples planning to have children can alert them to the possibility of their having a child with the disease. In addition, in utero testing for sickle cell disease can be done as early as the ninth week of pregnancy.

Where Can One Obtain More Information on Sickle Cell Anemia?

National Heart, Lung and Blood Institute
National Institutes of Health
Building 31, Room 4A21
Bethesda, MD 20892
(301) 496-4236

National Association for Sickle Cell Disease, Inc.
4221 Wilshire Blvd, Suite 360
Los Angeles, CA 90010
(213) 936-7205

Glossary

Chromosomes. Structures in the nucleus of the cell containing all of the genes arranged in a linear pattern

Gene. The unit of heredity; a segment of DNA that codes for the synthesis of a single protein

Hemoglobin. The chemical framework of the hemoglobin molecule that contains the iron atom and carries oxygen

Heterozygous. A condition in which there are two different genes at a given locus (place) on a pair of homologous (matched pair) chromosomes

Homologous. A matched pair; usually refers to chromosomes, one from each parent, having the same genes in the same order

Homozygous. A condition in which there are identical genes at a certain locus on homologous chromosomes

Locus. The position of a gene on a chromosome

Mutation. Change in the genetic code

Sources

National Heart, Lung, and Blood Institute
Center for Sickle Cell Disease, Howard University

Stroke

What Is Stroke?

A stroke is a cerebrovascular accident that occurs when part of the brain does not receive the flow of blood it needs. This happens when a blood vessel bringing oxygen and other nutrients to the brain bursts or is clogged by a blood clot. Because the nerve cells in the affected area of the brain are deprived of oxygen, they die within minutes. These nerve cells then permanently lose their ability to send messages to other parts of the body, resulting in such damage as partial paralysis, speech, language or memory loss, changes in behavior, and spatial and perceptual deficits.

What Are the Different Kinds of Stroke?

Cerebral thrombosis. This is the most common type of stroke. It occurs when a blood clot (thrombus) develops in an artery that is bringing blood to the brain. These clots are most likely to form in arteries already damaged by atherosclerosis.

Cerebral embolism. Between 5 and 14 percent of all strokes are caused by cerebral embolisms. This kind of stroke occurs when a wandering blood clot (embolism) that has been formed elsewhere is carried by the bloodstream to an artery either in the brain or leading to it.

Cerebral hemorrhage. About 10 percent of all strokes occur when blood from a burst artery goes directly into the brain. About half of these patients die, but the other half are likely to recover more fully than those who have had other kinds of stroke. Cerebral hemorrhage can be caused by a head injury or a burst aneurysm (a blood-filled pouch in a weak spot in an artery's wall).

Subarachnoid hemorrhage. Seven percent of strokes occur when a blood vessel on the brain's surface ruptures and bleeds into the space between the brain and the skull.

What Are the Risk Factors for Stroke?

High blood pressure. The American Heart Association states that high blood pressure is the most important risk factor for stroke. Many experts think that increased control of high blood pressure is the reason that the death rate from stroke dropped over 36 percent between 1976 and 1985.

Heart disease. People with heart problems have more than double the risk of stroke. Stopping cigarette smoking and reducing levels of blood cholesterol, in addition to controlling high blood pressure, greatly reduce the risk of both heart disease and stroke.

High red blood cell count. Medical treatment can correct this thick blood condition, which increases the risk of blood clots.

Transient ischemic attacks. Known as TIAs, these brief ministrokes are thought to precede about 10 percent of strokes. They can usually be treated with drugs that prevent blood clots from forming.

Age. Although 29 percent of the people who have strokes each year are under age 65, the risk of stroke more than doubles with each decade after age 65.

Sex. Men have a 30 percent higher risk of stroke than women.

Race. Black Americans have a 60 percent higher risk of stroke than whites; this may be related to the greater incidence of high blood pressure in blacks.

Diabetes. People with diabetes, especially those who have high blood pressure, are at increased risk for stroke. Women with diabetes are at greater risk than men.

Prior stroke. A person who has had one or more strokes is many more times likely to have another than is a person who has never had a stroke.

Heredity. A family history of stroke increases the chances of having one.

Age-Adjusted Mortality Rates By State, 1980: Stroke in the Total Population, Ages 35-74.

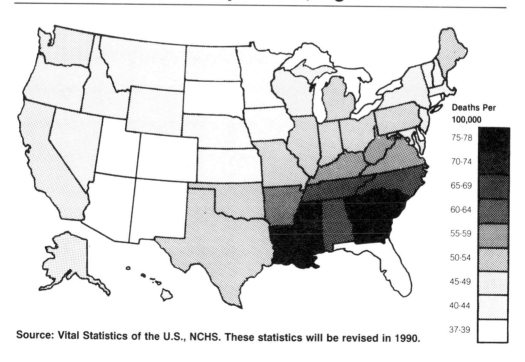

Deaths Per 100,000

75-78
70-74
65-69
60-64
55-59
50-54
45-49
40-44
37-39

Source: Vital Statistics of the U.S., NCHS. These statistics will be revised in 1990.

Percentage of Strokes Occurring in Various Age Groups

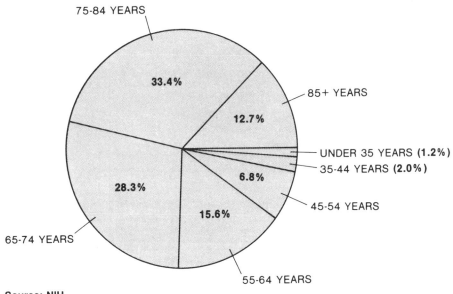

Source: NIH

Asymptomatic carotid bruit. The presence of an abnormal sound when a stethoscope is placed over the carotid artery, located in the neck, indicates an increased risk of stroke.

How Many Americans Have Strokes Each Year? How Many Die?

About 500,000 Americans have strokes each year, and in 1984, 155,000 died.

Half of all stroke patients are still alive 7 years later, but many do not fully recover. In one study, it was found that 31 percent of stroke survivors needed help caring for themselves, 20 percent needed help walking, and 71 percent had an impaired vocational capacity.

It is estimated that half of all patients hospitalized for acute neurologic diseases are stroke victims.

What Is the Cost of Stroke to Americans?

The American Heart Association has estimated the cost of stroke-related health care at $12.8 billion for 1987. This includes the total cost of health services, plus lost

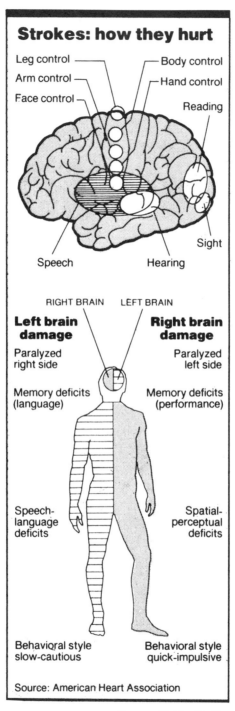

Bee graphic/Jim Chaffee

Source: The Sacramento Bee, September 15–October 3, 1985

productivity resulting from disability. Of the nearly 2 million Americans considered disabled from stroke, almost a third are wage earners aged 35 to 65 who have become unemployable because of their disability.

How Much Money Is Spent for Stroke-Related Research?

In 1987, the National Institute of Neurological and Communicative Disorders and Stroke will spend an estimated $26.5 million on stroke research. The National Heart, Lung, and Blood Institute allocated $11 million, for a total of $37.5 million.

What Advances Has Research Made in the Treatment and Prevention of Stroke in the Past 10 Years?

Many health professionals have credited the increase in control of high blood pressure for the 36 percent drop in the death rate due to stroke between 1976 and 1985. New drugs that provide effective control with fewer side effects have played a role in making this possible.

Better medical care of stroke victims has also contributed to reducing the death rate. Improved diagnostic technologies now allow identification of the section of the brain that has been damaged by stroke, and tests of blood flow can identify the location of blockages in the blood vessels. Drugs can be used to prevent additional blood clots from forming.

What Is the Outlook for Stroke?

Continued efforts to control risk factors for stroke—including high blood pressure and such factors as cigarette smoking and high blood cholesterol that put people at risk for heart disease—can be expected to further reduce the toll of stroke.

Where Can One Obtain More Information on Stroke?

National Institute of Neurological and Communicative Disorders
   and Stroke
National Institutes of Health
Building 31, Room 8A16
Bethesda, MD 20892
(301) 496-5924

American Heart Association
7320 Greenville Ave.
Dallas, TX 75231
(214) 750-5300

The Stroke Foundation
898 Park Ave.
New York, NY 10021
(212) 734-3434

Glossary

Aneurysm. Abnormal stretching or widening of a blood vessel wall; a ruptured aneurysm can cause a stroke

Embolus. Traveling blood clot that can plug a brain artery and cause a stroke

Hemorrhage. Loss of blood from a blood vessel; in external hemorrhage blood escapes from the body; in internal hemorrhage blood passes into tissues surrounding the ruptured blood vessel

Infarct. Mass of tissue consisting of a blood clot, dead nerve cells, and other debris that can block a blood vessel and cause a stroke

Thrombus. A clotted lump that forms within an artery, blocking blood flow

Transient ischemic attack (TIA). A brief ministroke caused by temporary blockage of a blood vessel

Sources

National Institute of Neurological and Communicative Disorders and Stroke
American Heart Association

Sudden Infant Death Syndrome

What Is Sudden Infant Death Syndrome?

The term sudden infant death syndrome (SIDS) is used to described the sudden and unexpected death of an apparently healthy infant. Crib death is also used to describe this tragedy. Medical scientists do not yet know what causes SIDS, but they have ruled out suffocation, choking, neglect, common infection, allergy, and reaction to immunizations.

Which Infants Appear Most Susceptible to SIDS?

A National Institute for Child Health and Human Development study of SIDS found that the peak incidence of SIDS was between the second and fourth months of life, and deaths were more likely to occur during cold weather months. The peak time of death was between midnight and 8 AM. Black infants were three times as likely to die of SIDS as whites, and infants born to teenage mothers and smokers were more likely to die of SIDS, as were babies who were premature and of low birth weight. Some researchers suggest that siblings of SIDS victims may be at increased risk; others disagree.

How Often Does SIDS Occur?

The National Institute of Child Health and Human Development estimates 7,000 deaths from SIDS each year. Ninety percent of these infants are under 6 months of age. SIDS is the leading cause of death of children between 1 and 12 months in the United States.

How Much Money Is Being Spent on SIDS Research?

The National Institute of Child Health and Development is spending $23.5 million on SIDS research during 1987 and plans to spend $23.6 million in 1988. The National Institute of Neurological and Communicative Disorders and Stroke has budgeted $2.5 million for each of these years.

What Advances in SIDS-Related Research Have Been Made in the Past 10 Years?

Research has not yet led to a cause or treatment for SIDS. However, investigations into SIDS continue, and knowledge of what happens when SIDS occurs is increasing.

Researchers have learned that there are changes in the brainstem tissues of SIDS infants and are now looking for cellular changes in this tissue. They also now know that there are small hemorrhagic spots on the lungs of SIDS victims.

A National Institutes of Health consensus panel has found evidence to be inconclusive for the value of electronically monitoring infants at home in the hope of preventing SIDS. These experts recommend the use of the monitors for only a small proportion of infants, even among those born prematurely or having brief episodes of apnea.

There are several organizations that offer help and counseling to parents who have lost infants to SIDS.

What Is the Outlook for SIDS?

The National Institutes of Health are supporting research studies that may show that SIDS is caused by a combination of deficiences in the newborn, resulting from the infant's failure to adapt to life outside the womb. Studies will attempt to characterize the specific immaturities thought to be involved in SIDS.

Where Can One Obtain More Information on SIDS?

National Institute of Child Health and Human Development
Office of Research Reporting
National Institutes of Health
Building 31, Room 2A04
Bethesda, MD 20892
(301) 496-5133

National Sudden Infant Death Syndrome Clearinghouse
8201 Greensboro Drive, Suite 600
McLean, VA 22102
(703) 821-8955

National Sudden Infant Death Syndrome Foundation
Metro Plaza Suite 104
8200 Professional Place
Landover, MD 20785
(301) 459-3388
1 (800) 221-SIDS

Glossary

Apnea. The absence of breathing
Crib death. A term used for sudden infant death syndrome
SIDS. Sudden infant death syndrome

Sources

National Sudden Infant Death Syndrome Foundation
National Institute of Child Health and Human Development

Trauma

What Is Trauma?

Trauma is the medical term for an injury, ranging from a small abrasion to a major injury.

What Are the Major Causes of Trauma?

Motor vehicle accidents. Motor vehicle accidents are the leading cause of accidental death. Crashes on public roads cause between 45,000 and 53,000 deaths each year and between 4 and 5 million injuries. The greatest number of motor vehicle fatalities in 1983 were 19-year-olds.

Falls. Falls are the second leading cause of unintentional death in the U.S. for people ages 45 to 74 and the first cause of accidental death for people 75 years and over. In 1984, 11,937 people died from falls.

Drowning. Drowning rates are highest among children 4 years and younger and for people 15 to 24 years of age. Eighty-four percent of all drowning victims are males.

Burns. Two people die every hour from burns. Each week, over 19,000 burn injuries occur, with 2,600 requiring hospitalization. The victim's own actions cause 75 percent of all burns; this increases to 81 percent of burns in people over age 70.

High school sports. Each year, about 800,000 high school athletes are injured, 100,000 of them seriously enough to prevent them from participation in games or practices for at least 3 weeks. The number of paralyzing injuries and deaths directly related to high school football is four times higher than for college and professional football combined.

All-terrain vehicles. In the first 9 months of 1985, there were 78,000 emergency room visits resulting from ATV accidents. When deaths occurred from these accidents, they were due to head and cervical spine injuries, neck fractures, internal organ injuries, and lung and chest injuries.

Firearms. Guns rank third, after motor vehicles accidents and falls, as a cause of spinal injuries.

Occupational injury on the job. Every year, about 2 million workers receive disabling injuries on the job. About 70,000 of these people become permanently impaired, and 11,600 die from their injuries.

How Many Americans Sustain Trauma Each Year? How Many Die?

The American Trauma Society states that every year 60 million people are traumatized in some way. As a result, nearly 9 million Americans are temporarily disabled, and 340,000 receive some form of permanent disability, including lost limbs, sight, or mobility. About 150,000 Americans die from trauma each year.

What Is the Cost of Trauma to This Country?

Trauma costs Americans $107.3 billion each year in lost wages, medical expenses, insurance administration costs, property damage, and indirect costs. More than $31.2 billion is lost in wages because trauma often affects people during or near the beginning of their most productive work years.

Trauma patients accumulate 19 million hospital days per year and total 7 million physician contacts for their care.

How Much Money Is Spent on Trauma Research Each Year?

The Committee on Trauma Research of the National Research Council and the Institute of Medicine found that, in 1983, the federal government spent $112 million for non-military research on the cause and prevention of injuries plus acute and long-term care and rehabilitation of the injured. This includes money spent by the National Institutes of Health and Centers for Disease Control, plus such other agencies as the Consumer Product Safety Commission, National Highway Traffic Safety Administration, Federal Aviation Administration, Federal Highway Administration, Coast Guard, Veterans Administration, Health Resources and Services Administration, and National Institute of Handicapped Research.

What Have Researchers Learned in the Past 10 Years About the Prevention of Trauma?

Collection of data on the causes of injury allows epidemiologists and other researchers to see accident patterns that can lead to preventive efforts. Mandatory seatbelt and child restraint laws and raising the drinking age to 21 are having an effect on the number of deaths and the severity of injury from motor vehicle accidents in some states. The American Trauma Society estimates that the use of smoke detectors cuts the risk of fire deaths in half.

Research on the care of trauma victims has led to improved training for emergency medical personnel. Advances in acute medical treatment and rehabilitation care increase the likelihood of recovery from trauma.

Leading causes of accidental death by age

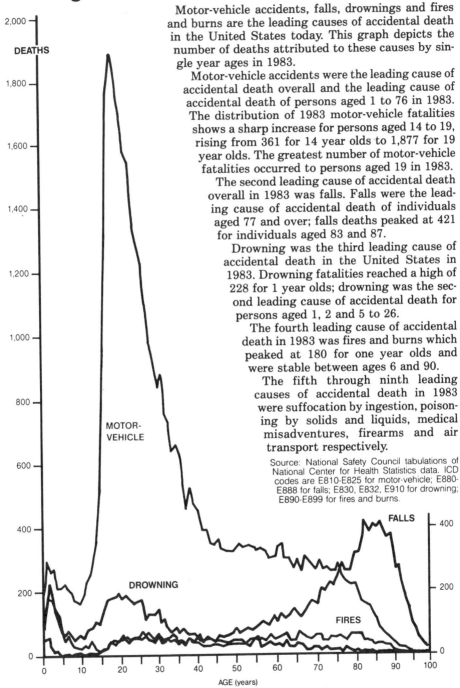

Motor-vehicle accidents, falls, drownings and fires and burns are the leading causes of accidental death in the United States today. This graph depicts the number of deaths attributed to these causes by single year ages in 1983.

Motor-vehicle accidents were the leading cause of accidental death overall and the leading cause of accidental death of persons aged 1 to 76 in 1983. The distribution of 1983 motor-vehicle fatalities shows a sharp increase for persons aged 14 to 19, rising from 361 for 14 year olds to 1,877 for 19 year olds. The greatest number of motor-vehicle fatalities occurred to persons aged 19 in 1983.

The second leading cause of accidental death overall in 1983 was falls. Falls were the leading cause of accidental death of individuals aged 77 and over; falls deaths peaked at 421 for individuals aged 83 and 87.

Drowning was the third leading cause of accidental death in the United States in 1983. Drowning fatalities reached a high of 228 for 1 year olds; drowning was the second leading cause of accidental death for persons aged 1, 2 and 5 to 26.

The fourth leading cause of accidental death in 1983 was fires and burns which peaked at 180 for one year olds and were stable between ages 6 and 90.

The fifth through ninth leading causes of accidental death in 1983 were suffocation by ingestion, poisoning by solids and liquids, medical misadventures, firearms and air transport respectively.

Source: National Safety Council tabulations of National Center for Health Statistics data. ICD codes are E810-E825 for motor-vehicle; E880-E888 for falls; E830, E832, E910 for drowning; E890-E899 for fires and burns.

Source: Accidents Facts, 1986 Edition. National Safety Council

What Is the Outlook for Trauma?

The American Trauma Society believes that not enough attention is paid to the care of trauma victims. Only 10 percent of American communities have effective trauma systems, with many trauma victims dying needlessly after they have reached the hospital because of lack of appropriate care.

The American Trauma Society states that if existing information about preventive measures were applied, the rate of trauma could be reduced by 50 percent and, with appropriate research and improved emergency medical services delivery, 25 percent of those who now die of injuries could be saved.

Where Can One Obtain More Information on Trauma?

American Trauma Society
P.O. Box 13526
Baltimore, MD 21203
(301) 328-6304

American College of Emergency Physicians
P.O. Box 619911
Dallas, TX 75261-9911
(214) 550-0911

Glossary

Epidemiologist. A specialist in the study of the prevalence and spread of disease and disability in a community
Paralysis. Loss of power of voluntary movement in a muscle through injury or disease
Rehabilitation. Development of a person's ability to function at optimum level
Triage. Medical screening of patients to determine their priority for treatment

Source

American Trauma Society

About the Editor

Terry L. Lierman is president of Capitol Associates, Inc., a Washington, D.C., government relations and consulting firm that encompasses the broad spectrum of health care. Mr. Lierman has had extensive experience in this field since 1972, when he began his career at the National Institutes of Health (NIH). His career has included the positions of Staff Director, Committee on Appropriations, and Staff Director, Subcommittee on Labor, Health and Human Services, and Education Appropriations. He is a frequent speaker on the issues of health care, particularly as they relate to government policy, and has developed a far-reaching network in both the private and public sector that is concerned with all aspects of the nation's health.